PROUDFLESH

Proudflesh

P. J. Worrell

thistledown press

Thistledown Press Ltd.
410 2nd Avenue North
Saskatoon, Saskatchewan, S7K 2C3
www.thistledownpress.com

Library and Archives Canada Cataloguing in Publication

Worrell P. J., 1949-, author
Proudflesh / P.J. Worrell.

Short stories.
Issued in print and electronic formats.
ISBN 978-1-927068-95-3 (pbk.).—ISBN 978-1-77187-002-3 (html).—
ISBN 978-1-77187-003-0 (pdf)

I. Title.

PS8645.O724P76 2014   C813'.6   C2014-900743-4
C2014-900744-2

Cover and book design by Jackie Forrie
Printed and bound in Canada

Canada Council   Conseil des Arts   SASKATCHEWAN   Canadian   Patrimoine
for the Arts   du Canada   ARTS BOARD   Heritage   canadien

Thistledown Press gratefully acknowledges the financial assistance of
the Canada Council for the Arts, the Saskatchewan Arts Board, and the
Government of Canada through the Canada Book Fund for its publishing
program.

PROUDFLESH

For my sister-in-law,
Lesley,

Love,
Peggy

For my sister, Marlene Montford,
and my brother, Howard Weinmaster

Contents

Asters

RACHEL IS ON ONE KNEE AT the front door tying her laces when she hears them come in from the garage and set down heavy bags, probably groceries, on the kitchen counter. David brings the carseat into the living room. Lilia is making snuffly piggy noises.

"Mother, could you take Lilia for a walk while we fix dinner?" Obviously they had planned this on the drive home.

"But I was just about to go for my run," she says over her shoulder, then stands up and stretches her back. "Oh, I suppose I could. I want to check out the autumn flora. I'll run in the morning instead."

"I noticed some scraggly asters. We've had a touch of frost." David is dressing Lilia in a red sweater no doubt knit painstakingly by the other grandmother. Her arms resist being forced into the sleeves. "The daycare said Lilia was fussy. It's her teeth."

"You cut your teeth without any problems."

"She has all of the symptoms," Avery interjects from the kitchen, like it's the second verse of a duet. *It's her teeth, it's her teeth.*

The third verse is David's. "She's had a hard time with every one of her teeth. Fever. Diarrhea. Poor thing."

Avery chimes in on the refrain. "It's her teeth". At least they're in harmony.

The First Year, with a pediatrician's endorsement, lies on the coffee table.

"Dave, give your mother one of those teething rings in the freezer." *Your mother.*

The decor is minimalist. Sleek white in contrast with rosewood floors. David scoots into the kitchen and returns with a nubbly lifesaver.

"You've been on the Koroluk Trail before. It's paved."

"I remember."

He prods Lilia's lips, but her tongue keeps thrusting the teething ring out, so he leaves it on her chest. His hair is thinning at the crown just like Gord's at the same age.

"Behind the condo construction site, you'll come to a fork," he says. "Veer to the left and take the gravel trail overlooking the river. It's picturesque."

"Okay."

"You'll see what I mean."

What a procedure, snapping the car seat into the stroller. David would have been meticulous in his analysis of the consumer research. Lilia screams when he fastens the straps. Rachel half-expects him to give a demonstration of its features. "Is she ready?"

"Yep. Would you mind taking Bono along?"

Avery is opening and closing cupboard doors. She calls out, "He won't be any bother."

"Fine."

Bono yips and bounces in anticipation. David puts him in a headlock to hook the leash onto his collar. "Now you behave for Grandma," he says. "Bags for his waste are in this pouch. They're biodegradable. Thanks Mom. It'll give Avery and me a little couple time. Just so you know, it's not safe to run with a stroller."

Rachel has been sequestered in David's house all day marking exams. She reaches the Koroluk Trail in a matter of minutes. The trees are alive with songbirds, each trying to upstage the other. Bono lifts his leg, releasing a cascade of acrid urine on the first pine. Runners and cyclists pass. Bono heels, his hot breath penetrating Rachel's running pants.

Couple time. Thirty years ago, she and Gord were as horny as a pair of spruce grouse. She'd be folding diapers on their second-hand couch with David on the floor, immersed in Mr. Rogers' Neighborhood. Gord was supposed to be studying at a card table in their bedroom. He'd appear, the crotch of his jeans bulging. They'd screw, facing the TV, with her on his lap in case David turned around. Mr. Rogers would hang his suit jacket in the closet, zip up a Perry Como cardigan over his shirt and tie, remove his dress shoes and put on sneakers. He'd sing, "*It's you I like, it's you yourself, it's you.*" He'd give them just enough time to grab a handful of Kleenex and pull up their pants. A domestic compromise.

The path winds through mixed boreal forest dominated by jack pine and white spruce. A chain blocks an offshoot winding downhill. "Soil erosion. Trail closed. Order #394".

"Good boy Bono." What a silly name for a dog.

She leans over the canopy to check on the baby, who has fallen asleep. Fine veins like blue threads are visible through her eyelids, the same as David's when Rachel used to breastfeed him. She would concentrate on his face, memorize his features. She couldn't get enough of him. She wanted to absorb him back into her womb, wanted David and her to become one again, to stay that way.

Will it be like this from now on? Grandmotherly duties foisted upon her and no time alone with her son? How she loved being with David when they were both single. They'd drink coffee and talk in their pyjamas for hours in the morning, go to bookstores and the opera, compete at Scrabble.

And then, "Mom, I would like you to meet Avery Popoff. We're both in Organic Chem. She's the smartest woman I've ever known." They held hands, they looked into each other's eyes, they smooched. Then there was the wedding with Rachel and Gord sitting together at the head table, dancing on cue, pretending to be a couple. After all, they were the parents of the groom.

Bono stalls and squats, back arched. No way she's picking up dog crap. It's in the understory of the jack pines anyway, in the jumble of seedlings and native flora.

Frost has caused the asphalt to heave and rupture in places. Rachel slows her pace so the series of protuberances won't rouse Lilia. A thirty-something runner, male, overtakes her. Then two women attempting a short-of-breath conversation. "He just doesn't get it," one says, and the other replies, "Eugene doesn't either."

She rotates her head to relieve the numbness in her neck. If only she were on her mountain bike ascending the Grouse Grind.

And then there was the big announcement. "*We're* pregnant." Those were David's words on the phone, and what could she say? "Congratulations! I'm so happy for you."

She made the mistake of telling one of her colleagues. A few weeks before Avery (or would it be David *and* Avery?) gave birth, her admin assistant had interrupted, insisting she come to the staff lounge at coffee time. She had been scrambling to meet the submission deadline for *The Canadian Journal of Botany*. They sat her in a rocking chair, made her put on a grey Mrs. Claus wig with a bun, and arranged knitting needles in her hands. She smiled for the photo, laughed along when they presented the plastic potty with chunks of wieners set in yellow Jello. Then there was cake. She wanted to say, "Don't you people have any work to do?"

And here she is, pushing a baby stroller. The chill in the air and the diversity of plant life please her. She keeps her eyes peeled for her precious asters. Bono pays no heed to a pair of crows perched on an anthill made of pine needles. City employees have sawn deadfall into two-foot lengths, possibly for firewood. So far, she has seen only a few silvery flashes of the river through the trees.

An elderly couple, arm in arm, stop to admire Lilia. "What a darling," the woman coos. "Grandchildren are such a blessing, aren't they?"

"Mmm hmm." What can Rachel do except smile in concordance with this universal truth? No one has spoken the word "blessing" to her since her wedding. "Dear God, Bless this young couple . . . blah blah blah."

The construction site. The fork. David said to turn left.

Coniferous trees give way to quaking aspen *Populus tremuloides*. The rise in elevation makes it challenging for Rachel to navigate the stroller on gravel. Corded roots of aspens undulate across the path. This might not be a work-out, but her heart rate must be up to 100 BPM.

Can that pungent scent be sagebrush? In an open area, sure enough she spots the blue-green blur. First Peoples used the seeds for food and the plant for a fire-starter. She is surprised it grows this far north. Overhead a nuthatch is sending out its tin-fluty call notes.

To propel the stroller up the incline, Rachel has to lock her elbows. She pauses on a craggy precipice over a ravine that deepens dramatically. A draft catches Bono's slobber and swings it onto her pantleg, leaving a glistening smear on the black Spandex. White paper bark on birch saplings dot a collage of elderberry and honeysuckle. The river is fifty feet below. Elijah Blue grass *Festuca glauca* must have escaped from someone's garden. When David was in grade two, she wrote her dissertation on the introduction of Blue fescue to western Canada.

She has been so engaged in surveying plant life on the downward slope that she has failed to notice the vista. "Picturesque indeed," she says out loud when the blaze of golds, oranges, and reds on the opposite bank come to her awareness. The colours cue a memory of the Cape Breton Highlands one October when she was invited to present a paper at the annual meeting of the Botanical Association in Halifax, then rented a car and toured the Cabot Trail by herself. Gord had accompanied her to Halifax. They had tickets for the Celtic Colours Festival, but he took an early flight home after a blow-out at the hotel. Six months later, he moved from Vancouver to Calgary.

The wind gusts above the broad river valley. A red-headed pileated woodpecker drums on a rotting stump, mining for its supper. Surely the path will loop back any time. Mmm . . . Spiked Muhly Grass *Muhlenbergia glomerata*. What was the name of the Alberta botanist who first detected hybridization with Green Muhly? Van or Vander . . . something. He insisted there was no need to differentiate the two species, but Rachel held firm to the position that they be treated separately based on cytological, morphological, and ecological differences.

She peeks into the stroller. The teething ring is defrosting on Lilia's sweater. Rachel breathes in sweet baby smell and puts the useless thing in a storage pouch. Lilia has inherited that appealing combination of dark hair, a fair complexion, and blue eyes from Gord. (David's referring to him as "Granpa Gord".) Rachel is softened by the child's dimpled chin, no bigger than a *birch bolete* mushroom. Her index finger musters the nerve to reach in and stroke Lilia's chubby little hands, soft as marshmallows. She brushes her lips across the fine baby hair. Fortunately Lilia doesn't take after Avery's side of the family, those long narrow Popoff faces, the incisors of a rodent.

A pair of grey squirrels is playing chase in two lone spruce trees, up one trunk and down the other. That is, until they spot Bono. They retreat to the highest branches, boldly squeaking and scolding from a position of safety. Bono rears up and yelps, strangling himself. Rachel jerks him back, and blurts out, "Stop it. Don't be a pain in the butt." A magpie adds its voice to the reprimand. Lilia sleeps through the commotion.

The scents of Labrador tea and lichen are earthy and sharp. The path narrows. It becomes too narrow for the stroller's two rear wheels. Rachel has to tip up the left side like mowing the lawn on a slope, except the stroller has three wheels instead of four. Plus the weight of the baby. Rachel's trainers sink into a spongy carpet of sphagnum moss. Cool wetness seeps through her soles. They should've closed off this section. Maybe it's just a short stretch. What was David thinking when he recommended this trail? The construction site was dormant, she recalls.

Mammoth machines stuck in mud up to their axles. The workers must have been sent home.

Bono hangs back. The loop of his leash is around Rachel's right wrist. She tries to roll the stroller in reverse, but the rear wheels refuse to budge in the quagmire. Lilia stirs, flings one plump little fist out to each side. Rachel's temples are throbbing and the back of her neck is damp. It's a goddam bog! No wonder she hasn't encountered another human being since the fork. The sun dips below the horizon, imbuing the river valley with a mellow aura. David will remind Avery that his mother is a fitness fanatic most likely circumambulating the city with Lilia. Acid reflux burns Rachel's esophagus. Her shoes are drenched. That's when the Alberta botanist's name comes to her — Vanderhof.

She stops to collect her thoughts. She could carry Lilia. To Hell with the eco green stroller. But she can't reach the baby from the back because of the canopy and there is no room to get around to the front. Bono pokes his muzzle into the back of her knee. She considers freeing him, but what if he hurdles forward and pushes the stroller sideways to the left? Her predicament is unfathomable in a yuppie neighbourhood within walking distance of downtown. "Stay calm," she tells herself. She tries relaxation breathing, deliberates, then pushes on, leaning to her right to balance the stroller on one rear wheel, just inching along. She can feel the strain in her arms and her back despite her level of fitness. On her fortieth birthday, she began the regimen of early morning work-outs at the gym, running, and cycling. The payoff has been a fifty pound weight loss and the satisfaction of fitting into Size Zero clothing.

Jesus Christ. Her feet slither in dead plant matter, muskeg concealed by late afternoon shadows. Bono is getting antsy. She allows his leash to slip off her hand and pushes him hard to the right with her calf. "Take off." When he just stands there, she kicks him with the toe of her wet sneaker and hollers, "Go on, you stupid animal!" He bounds up the hill dragging his leash and provokes the wrath of the squirrels once again. Now Rachel's only responsibility is Lilia, who is awake and whimpering.

Fuck. The stroller slides sideways at an angle. She doesn't have the strength to keep it upright. She loses her footing in ooze and lands on her ass, hard, but hangs onto the stroller. They are on their way down.

Thorns of rose bushes prick her neck, conglomerate rock scrapes her arms, roots exposed by soil erosion jar her spine. She grips the handlebar with every one of her knuckles. When the stroller bounces over stones, Lilia bawls. At least she is protected by the thick padding, shoulder straps, and seatbelt.

They land on rocks in icy ankle-deep water, scaring a flock of Canada geese into flight. Far-off sewage pong blends with a fresh breeze. Rachel clambers to her feet and tries to right the stroller, but the frame has twisted and the thing is off-balance with its front wheel and one of its rear wheels in the water, the other on the shoreline. Lilia is wailing. She must be lying on her side. Unable to secure her footing in the crevices between slippery stones, Rachel wobbles. Water washes over her feet. The handlebar slips out of her numb hands. She is able to touch it with her fingertips, but can't get a hold. She tiptoes gingerly from one stone to the next until the water is waist-deep. With both arms, she grapples the lopsided stroller again and again, but each time it slips out of her hands. Lilia must be wet by now.

The current is carrying the stroller away. Rachel thrashes, and grasps at nothing.

The stroller disappears. Rachel plunges in headfirst, but can't see it through the churned-up water. She attempts the breast-stroke, but tall weeds wind around her legs, hobbling her. She manages to free herself and crawl to shore. She stands up in heavy wet clothing and waves both arms above her head like the survivor of an airplane crash in the Arctic. The current is flowing in the direction of the bridge. She yells for help even though no one can possibly hear her over the whoosh of the river and the hum of rush hour traffic on the bridge.

She screams, "LILIA!"

The stroller surfaces, bobbing on its side. With her knees high, Rachel marches into the river in pursuit, but the ruthless current keeps knocking her off her feet. The stroller flips rightside up and travels down the middle of the river as if pushed by an apparition. Rachel attempts giant steps synchronized with the current, but is swept forward and pulled under. She resurfaces, stands, and can only watch the stroller speed up and do somersaults. It's like a convertible in a carwash, top down, windows open, water flooding in, the driver's seatbelt fastened.

"DAVID!" It was his idea, the walk.

Rachel catches a whiff of diesel. She pukes. She coughs. She pukes some more. She reaches out in front, both arms perpendicular to her body. A futile reach. The outline of the stroller blurs, the green of it blending with the brown water and the white froth and the shiny rocks. One brief patch of red.

Lilia is gone.

The bent toe of one of Rachel's shoes is wedged under a rock. She shifts her weight to the other foot flat in saturated silt. She lets her arms drop to her sides. From the waist down, she is numb. From the waist up, she is catatonic.

She remembers falling in love with David, skin to skin in the postpartum recovery room. And the ceremony honouring her with the President's Medal in Science, the cornflower blue ribbon being looped over her head.

The landscape transforms into the painting on the wall of her office. *Autumn.* Acrylic on canvas by Ken Christopher. The slope above her is an insipid palette — browns, greens, and golds — birch saplings stripped bare against a dusky sky. But the distant riverbank. . . . "Oh," she gasps. Vibrant reds, tender mauves, profound purples in solidarity with black, leaving no space for neutral, no cubbyhole for sad, no fissure for pride. The colours soak in and dye her.

She shifts her eyes from the horizon to the river. Not the sunset, not the bridge, not even the plant life, only the river, the hungry river. She holds her mind to the grey-brown concentric lines splashing over and around rocks, finding their way, refusing to be impeded. She is no longer in her intellect, she is in her core. Nothing will stop those lines from barrelling downstream, droning, frantic.

She cannot bear to tell David, to witness the horror on his face. Fatherhood becomes him. He dotes on Lilia, calls her his angel. Rachel's only choice is to dive in, to gulp the filthy river water and inhale it through her nose. There is no flailing.

A clown breathes into one balloon, twists the end into a knot, and offers it to Rachel. A yellow orb, a memory — a scorching California afternoon, a concrete sidewalk, black ants ten times the size of those back home. Rachel and her cousin Joanne are burning the ants with a magnifying glass. It was Joanne's idea. One of the ants bites Rachel's left thumb. The clown reaches into his pocket and tosses out other balloons, but they fall to the ground, no more than dabs of colour. Murky water fills her lungs. She won't fight her way to the surface. She won't be rescued by a marathon runner scrambling down from the path or a heroic CEO in a suit leaping from the bridge.

The cousins relish their sordid science experiment. Rachel sucks her ant bite. Joanne positions her index fingers at the corners of her eyes, hooks her baby fingers into the corners of her mouth, and stretches her face like pull taffy. Rachel giggles so hard she pees her pants.

Goldie's Tumour

MARTIN IS HEADED WEST ON THE Number 1 back to Calgary. He's half-listening to Q107 and picturing some guy porking Lenore. The image makes his back arch and his right foot flex up off the gas pedal. A transport truck passes him, then a fancy RV.

A green and white sign reads "Kildare 1 km". He makes a spur-of-the-moment decision, touches the brake, switches lanes, makes a left turn, crosses the divided highway, and bumps across railroad tracks on a narrow gravel road.

Three farm trucks are angle-parked in front of Debbie's Country Café with "OPEN" flashing in red neon. New Horizons for Seniors is next door, and across the street is Propp's Foodeteria. Martin burns a Uey, parks, opens his car door, dumps a styrofoam cup of sunflower seed shells, gets out. The businesses on either side of the grocery store are boarded up.

If Martin's parents were alive, he'd ask them, "What were you thinking, bringing up five boys in the armpit of Saskatchewan?" One of the armpits. Maybe they'd say they got stuck in Kildare with its one grocery store, one café, one school, one church. One-of-each-ville. More like nothing-ville.

A piece of paper is taped to the glass door of Propp's Foodeteria. "Closing for good on March 16. Everything ½ price". That's today. Martin hasn't been in the store since he was seventeen years old and he has shown up on the exact day it's closing. The coincidence pisses him off. Alongside grocery carts in the porch is a bulletin board. "Will do spring cleaning" "Puppies to give away" "Bull sale". He opens the second glass door and walks into his childhood.

A zitty teenage cashier looks up from *People* magazine and forces a smile. Martin clears his throat. A woman in an office is shuffling a slough of papers on her desk. He walks down one aisle, then up another. It's like viewing a body before the burial. The merchandise on the rusted white metal shelves is sparse — canned peas, shaving cream, strawberry jam. The swinging doors at the back are like the saloon in Gunsmoke. His stomach cramps at the sight of those doors.

This used to be Glickmans' Fine Foods. Martin was neither proud of his parents owning a store nor was he embarrassed. It was simply *the store*. "Where's Mum?" "She's at *the store*." It was normal, until he left home that is, and found out about people with weekends off, season tickets for the Stampeders, and a time-share in Florida.

Sundays were the only days the store was closed (but Martin's old man still had to go down to check in case the power had gone off). Shabbat was supposed to be from sundown on Friday to sundown on Saturday, but Saturday was the busiest day at the store, so the Glickmans had to observe Shabbat a day late. Martin's father would recite some prayers. His mother would light two candles and, if she wasn't exhausted, bake two loaves of braided bread.

When Martin's youngest brother Goldwyn was in grade five, his mother noticed a lump on the side of his neck. She figured it must be his thyroid. When it thickened to the size of a hamburger patty, she took him to the doctor in Swift Current who advised against operating in case *it* spread throughout his body. Goldie kept on doing what ten-year-old boys do until he couldn't wear pullovers or turn his head to one side anymore. By then, the lump had sprouted wiry black hairs. A specialist in Saskatoon called it a malignant mass on his carotid artery and said it would eventually block his esophagus and windpipe and shut down his hearing.

Martin is looking at a tub of Cool Whip in the freezer, but what he's seeing is Goldie with his neck wrapped in a bandage, stepping down off the bus with Mum. After the operation, they gave Goldie ten years. It's hard to say how close they were.

A person feels shamed into buying something in a store that's going belly-up, but what? A can of luncheon meat past its expiry date? A dog-eared birthday card? Martin picks up a battered cardboard box of white emergency candles. Six inches long. Could they possibly be from when his parents owned the store? Could they have doubled as menorah candles? During Hanakkah, his mother used to light a menorah on their windowsill, one candle the first night, two the second, and so on up to eight (just in case there was anybody who didn't already know they were Jewish). Kildare was a typical prairie town. A Chinaman owned the café and a Jew owned the store.

Martin tries to stifle his cough as he approaches the check-out. The woman from the office, presumably the owner, is going over an invoice with the cashier. He offers his condolences and pays for the candles. The woman shrugs. Her pendulous breasts do a little shimmy. "Yeah, there's been a grocery store in town for almost fifty years." She's looking at the logo on his shirt pocket, "Bernard Misky's Restaurant Equipment and Supplies" with a screen-printed picture of BM. Martin sucks in his gut. She continues, "But people are fickle. They're doing their shopping at the Superstore or Costco in Medicine Hat."

"Yeah?"

"We lost the bank, then the post office, now the store."

"You retiring?"

"Nope." She's full of beans now. "It's time for a career change. I'm taking the Home Care Aide course at the community college in Swift Current in September. It'll be a blast."

He nods. His mother would've been good at looking after old people, but *career change* wasn't in her vocabulary. He has no clue if she worked full-time in the store or whether she stayed at home until the boys started school, like Lenore did. And what about summer holidays? Some more questions he never got around to asking.

He feels an urge to check out the back of the store. "Do you spose I could use your washroom?"

The owner points toward the back. "Through the doors and to the left."

By the time he separates the swinging doors, he's short of breath and his temples are throbbing. There's nothing familiar, just some boxes and a trolley. After school, the five Glickman boys used to elbow their way in from the back alley through the freight door. There was a yellow chrome set with four chairs, a tweed davenport, and a little black-and-white TV. His mother would have lunch set out — buttered buns, garlic sausage, a package of broken cookies, a dented can of juice and some glasses. It was musical chairs with one of them left standing, usually Goldie. They were animals, reaching over each other, grabbing food and stuffing it in their mouths. The old man had trained them to stay in the back. If they noticed him peering over the swinging doors, they knew they had better tone it down or else.

The bathroom is so small that Martin has to flatten his back against the wall to swing the door closed. He coughs up a ball of phlegm and spits it into the toilet, sits down. The sink is chipped, there's a build-up of grunge along the baseboards. He takes a shit, washes up with a bar of Lifebuoy with long dark crevices, sprays lilac air freshener, and leaves the door ajar.

There used to be a butcher block back here. His father would cut up meat and his mother would wrap the chunks in waxed brown paper, slap on wet brown tape, tie the parcels with string, and stamp them "Roast", "Soup Bones", "Steak", "Stew". Martin is borderline turned-on being back here, kinda like when Sarisons leave him a key to check their condo while they're down south.

Martin's mother grew up in the back of a butcher shop. Her father didn't adhere to Kosher slaughtering rules because all of their customers were Gentile. She told Martin and Goldie about one butchering day when her brother Charlie was outside playing with miniature farm implements in the dirt. She was shelling peas on the step and saw, and heard it all, the steer bucking and bawling in the holding chute, Charlie covering his ears, the gunshot, her father slitting the steer's throat, blood spurting all over him. Her Uncle Albert helped her father behead the animal, gut it, cut off its tail, and skin it. They rolled the carcass onto a canvas tarp and dragged it into the shop. Her father stayed inside. Uncle Albert was in charge of clean-up. He filled a wheelbarrow with remains and hauled them to the burning pit, then came back to load up the rest. He plunked the steer's head on top.

Charlie was stirring up little clouds of dust with his toy tractor. Uncle Albert stopped next to him, picked up the bloody head with its eyes bulging and arteries dripping, and lifted it into the air with both hands. He imitated the sound of the steer bawling before it was shot.

Martin can see his mother's face. She is telling him and Goldie the story of the uncle they would never meet. She stretches out the word *bawl*. Her lips are parted and her mouth curves downward on both sides when she says Uncle Albert "bawled just like the steer." She re-enacts setting down the pail of peas on the step, standing up, leaning forward and reaching out to her brother. "Come here Charlie. Hurry!" Uncle Harold chased him partway, then turned around laughing and put the head back in the wheelbarrow. Charlie was a frail and timid little boy, she said, and after that he never spoke another word. Goldie echoed her. "Never spoke another word." Eventually Charlie was labelled *retarded* and sent to an institution in North Battleford. Martin remembers his mother taking the bus to visit him. She was gone overnight.

What used to be a walk-in meat cooler is now a storage room. The abattoir would deliver freshly slaughtered cattle or pigs and hang them in the cooler to age. There was only one time Martin was ever alone in the store. It was a Sunday afternoon and his mother had sent him for a pound of margarine because they were having corn on the cob for supper. He dared himself to go into the cooler where a pig carcass was barely discernible in the dim light. He double-checked to make sure the heavy door wouldn't swing closed behind him, then stepped in. It couldn't be any worse than the umpteen times Pete, Dave, and Luke scared the bejeesus out of him.

The smell of raw meat and the pool of blood on the cement floor made his little peeny wriggle. He went up close and pretended the flesh marbled with yellow fat was a girl's thing. He slid his jeans and underwear partway down and out sprung his cocktail sausage. He touched the tip of it against the cold pig and kept on pressing until a spot warmed up and dented in. He had never seen a girl's privates, only the diagram in the Encyclopedia Britannica. He wouldn't find out about the hair until years later. His dink grew to the size of a breakfast sausage. Rubbing its head against those snaking veins made his vision go blurry. The carcass started to swing from the hook as if it were alive. It wasn't long until he let out a squeal no louder than a newborn kitten and a few droplets trickled on the floor. Halfway home, he remembered the margarine and had to run back to get it.

Here he stands with emergency candles in a plastic grocery bag. It will never be clearer than this. His old man's white apron is hanging on a nail beside the butcher block, spattered with blood. His mother is out front talking to a customer about rheumatism. He can hear her. "It's a good day when you wake up and your back doesn't give you no grief." Any minute, his brothers will burst through the door from the back alley.

Maybe Goldie would've turned out to be a pompous prick like Dave, Pete, and Luke. Or he might've been a softie like Martin's favourite Easter eggs, hard chocolate on the outside, marshmallow on the inside. He has stocked up on Easter eggs for the Stampeders' pre-season game, along with a 12-pack, pepperoni sticks, and chips. Maybe Martin and Goldie would've been buddies.

Goldie's tumour was the worst thing that could ever happen, or so they thought at the time. Ever since, there's been an invisible layer of shit floating over Martin's head like a threatening cloud. Sure it's invisible, but how can he relax when he know what's up there?

A yellow X-acto knife is lying with its blade exposed on a carton of No Name Toilet Tissue. He takes it into the bathroom, closes the door, and looks in the mirror. He hates his liver lips. Lenore used to nibble on the grey hair at his temples and whisper, "Yoohoo, Curlilocks. It's me, Goldilocks." It was her way of saying she was horny. Now she's shacked up on the weekends with some guy from the oil patch.

He cocks his head to one side, scrutinizes his neck, and with his index finger finds a bulging vein. This won't be the first time. He pokes the tip of the blade into his flesh until blood oozes out. He feels a little rush. He dabs blood with his finger, holds it to his nose and inhales. Blood trickles down his neck. He dabs again before it reaches his shirt collar, smears it on his tongue. If only he can smell and taste Glickman blood in this god-forsaken town, in this store that's closing for good. For Goldie.

Goldie died in a fight at a gravel pit party. No charges were laid. The coroner called it "teenage roughhousing".

Martin ignores his hard-on, presses a wad of toilet paper against the puncture hole in his neck, coughs, clears his throat, coughs some more. He's antsy now. If he's late returning the company car, BM will rag on him. There's a Walk-in Clinic on the way into Calgary on 17th. He should get his cough checked out, maybe have a chest X-ray. No, he'll have to wait until the hole heals up.

He's paranoid about his breathing and about every mole or pain. Lenore used to call him a hypochondriac. And he never even told her about the layer of shit floating over his head like a cloud. Dark. Foul. Vile. Without warning, it could squirt a drop of watery crap into his hair. He's always on edge, never carefree, not even for an instant. He has nightmares about a tsunami of turds knocking him down and burying him. Does everyone with cancer in their family have the same putrid layer over their heads? That would make for a sizeable build-up of stink and gloom in the world. It's gotta have some impact.

Change of Life

Proudflesh

Joy brought her sons home from the hospital to this blue bungalow. With a Sold sign on the front lawn, she is now free to go. A real estate agent chosen from the Yellow Pages closed the deal. She gave each of the boys a box of childhood mementos, whether he wanted them or not. The CMHA picked up the piano, extra furniture, and household items. She and Earl had accrued two or more of everything — fridges, rakes, colanders, Bibles, cats.

"Why do you want to live up there all by yourself?" each son, in his turn, asked. A reasonable question, Joy had to admit.

"Because I like the scents," she told Ross. "Rain. Wood smoke. Earth rot. The pine forest on a hot day."

To Billy she said, "Because of the changing of the seasons. I want to witness the performance."

And to AJ, "I'm learning about constellations and need dark sky."

What Joy didn't mention is that she is no longer fit to be seen in public. After meals, she has to check for a dry crust of milk at the corners of her mouth, or bread dough lodged between her front teeth like crack filler. Observing other women her age in church, she has learned not to run her fingers below her jawline, checking for sprouting hairs. Her double chin is threatening to triple, and she's growing a fleshy wattle.

She locks the door behind her, passes the weeping birch where her sons posed in rented tuxedos for their grad pictures, and drives away without looking back. Her destination is Otter Lake, the cabin she inherited from her parents. It will be a test of her mettle.

It is dark when she pulls up in the Merc loaded to the hilt. Almost all of the snow has melted. Jemima, her Boston terrier, bolts after being confined to the back seat with boxes and the cats, and runs laps around the yard. Joy looks up at the night sky. A lovely shiver begins in her ears and moves down her neck to her heart and stomach. With hands, one on top of the other on her chest, she inhales the scents of the North. The solitary listening and gathering period of her life will begin here at Otter Lake.

She sets down a bag of groceries and a container of water on the step and fumbles with the lock. The eavestroughs are dripping. Inside the closed-up cabin, the air is cold and dusty, with a hint of propane gas. The kitchen light and CBC Radio come on when she flips the breaker. Shelagh Rogers' laugh is a little fuzzy. She and Earl had to save up before they could afford to bring in the electricity.

She lights the pilot lights, fills the teakettle with water, and starts a fire in the pot-bellied stove in the living room. An antique mirror reflects her smile, the fire crackles, the kettle begins to sing.

Her hands smelling of Ivory soap, chamomile tea steeping in her grandmother's china cup, she settles into the La-Z-Boy.

The car can wait until tomorrow to be unpacked. Puffs of wood smoke from the stove reach her cool nose. She can envision Earl stretched out on the old tweed couch. The cats come in from the verandah and familiarize themselves with every nook, then clamor for body heat on her lap. "Girls, shoo!"

She scans the room — the rough wood slabs on the walls, the brown furniture, her mother's red-and-white gingham touches. It takes her back to her childhood, grumbling when she was expected to pump water and carry wood. Should she spiff the place up or leave it the way it is?

Carol Shields, Gabrielle Roy, Seán Virgo, Isak Dinesen — she has chosen her companions with deliberation. Her favourite CDs are stacked beside the stereo on an end table — Glenn Gould, Measha Brueggergosman, James Ehnes, a promising young tenor named Aaron Ferguson. She will listen to music, read, bake Health Bread with cranberries, and learn the origins of constellations in Greek mythology. After a lifetime of being awed by the night sky, she is able to identify only The Big Dipper and The Little Dipper.

If Henry David Thoreau, the grand-daddy of the Romantic Movement, communed with nature and pondered the essential meaning of life, why can't Joy? She will dabble in astronomy and observe sunsets in hopes of witnessing the rare green ray, that streak of light rising from the sun like a spurting fountain, throbbing, then disappearing.

There is nothing of any monetary value in the cabin, but everything has meaning to Joy — quilts her mother made for each of the boys, her father's bucksaw from the farm, the Mexican beach blanket they bought in California on Boxing Day, her snowshoes, the *Jaws* puzzle Earl laminated and hung in the boys' bedroom, her mother's cross-stitch: *Bless this house, O Lord we pray, Make it safe by night and day.*

The next morning, lying in bed in the half-darkness, Joy slips one hand under the elastic waist of her pyjama bottoms and rests it on a chubby thigh. Might a man be pleased by her plump parts? She remembers Earl saying, "Your li'l muffin smells sour tonight." His kisses were too soft, more like a woman's. She gets up to light a fire, then crawls back in between the flannelette sheets with the cats until the cabin warms up. Through the bedroom window, the sky lightens from black to blue-black, stars still visible. Here, the mornings come softly.

She tours the cabin in a terry cloth bathrobe and socks, looking out of the window in each room. Last night, she couldn't see the lake or the pine forest. Coffee tastes better at the cabin than anywhere else. Earl used to bring a cup to her in bed on Saturday mornings.

Pulling rumpled clothes out of a suitcase, she dresses, combs her hair and tucks it behind her ears, brushes her teeth, washes her face and smooths on Nivea Soft. She says out loud, "I don't give a rat's ass what I look like."

Outside, the air is crisp. At the lakeshore, Joy listens to the ice moaning. For the first time, she will be here to witness spring break-up, the grinding and roaring. There's a coating of frost on the windshield of the Merc. She carries in all the boxes. A bold Whiskey Jack swoops from pine branch to picnic table to pine branch, making its presence known, demanding a handout. She sets out breadcrumbs for the bird and brings in enough wood for one day, tracking in dirt and leaves, but not bothering to sweep.

Tea with honey, a eucalyptus candle, an open book in her hands, Jemima asleep at her feet, this is perfect, until the combined scents of bergamot and eucalyptus trigger a flashback to floral arrangements at Earl's funeral.

At the base of each pine tree, circles of exposed moss and low-bush cranberry increase in circumference daily as the remaining snow melts. In Earl's Size 12 rubber boots, Joy digs drainage ditches to hurry the run-off, rakes up the sodden birch leaves, feels the crunch of the old-man's-beard lichen, revels in the lime green buds as they open, and touches the soft needles on the tamaracks. Ah! Sun candles on the lake.

On her way out the door the cats always reach up and claw the knees of her pants. "You girls guard the cabin. C'mon Jemima, no moon tonight, it'll be pitch black." After three months at Otter Lake, this has become her bedtime ritual on clear nights — stargazing followed by a warm bath. When she pauses on the crude wooden bridge, it occurs to her that the creek trickles day and night whether she is paying attention or not.

In the mirror, her cheekbones are sharper. For forty years, she chose a hairstyle to conceal the craters of blackheads inside her ears, teenage zits impervious to squeezing with fingernails or gouging with a bobby pin. Here she boldly pushes her hair behind her ears (except when she's going to town for library books or to Digger's for milk).

She monitors the lengthening days, then stays up all night so she won't miss a minute of the longest day of the year. A clear sky sets the stage for breathtaking performances by satellites, meteors, and the Milky Way. She walks south, comes back for an intermission with popcorn and Fresca, walks north, then back home toward dawn for hot chocolate. She covers herself with a striped Hudson Bay blanket and lies back on a chaise lounge, watching the sun rise. A Summer Solstice party for one.

A faded newspaper clipping is stuck onto the mirror of her dresser with brittle scotch tape. "A real woman can hold down a full-time job, teach Sunday School, volunteer to chaperone her little darlings' field trips, keep the piano dusted, be an eager lover, and have the picnic basket packed and ready to go." The Women's Movement tried to convince Joy she could have it all — marriage, family, career, self-actualization. Bullshit.

Before leaving the city, she dropped off her fitted clothes, shoes with heels, and Earl's things in black garbage bags at the MCC Thrift Shop, and bought three sweatsuits at Walmart without trying them on. She looks at herself in the mirror. Her waist is thickening, she is becoming apple-shaped. She sings the chorus of *Waltzing with Bears*, sashaying and twirling in the narrow space between the dresser and the foot of her bed. Her neck looks sinewy, ropey when she sings. She's getting tough like a stewing hen, but her chins are soft and trembly. Next time she goes to town, she'll have to put on makeup and a bra so they can't say she's let herself go.

After breakfast most days, she feeds the Whiskey Jack raisins from her hand, then canoes to the beach with Jemima, a blanket, a towel, and her lunch. She curls her toes into the cool, damp sand, and flips through a magazine or dozes. The boys used to collect rocks or dig holes to China, even though they knew the holes would fill with water. How many goddamn bloodsuckers did they squish with rocks? Should she have stopped them?

On rainy days, she teaches herself the pieces in her *Book of Celtic Songs for Beginner Violin* — *My Luve Is Like A Red, Red*

Rose. Pretty Peggy. Hard is my Fate. Back in the city, when piano music sounded funereal to her ear, she bought a violin over eBay for two hundred dollars. In her obituary, they can say she "took up the violin after her husband's death, to fill in the gap."

Billy, Ross, Cheryl, and the children visit the first week in July. The houseful delights Joy. She has missed family, yet is growing to treasure solitude. Until the fifteenth of July, the day she disrupts her routine, the Otter Lake chapter in her life has been blissful. She sets out for a load of firewood from a sawmill, pulling a trailer Earl crafted from the amputated rear end of a half-ton truck, a royal blue GMC. She phoned ahead to order a half-cord of seasoned birch and poplar from a man with a Scottish burr. How did a Scot end up in northern Saskatchewan?

The Merc shimmies along a sandy road cut through bush leading to a ranch-style gate branded with a Celtic cross. A cluster of buildings is in view, plus heavy equipment and heaps of timber. This must be McPherson's Crossing. "For shit's sake, what is this?" Shanties in a row, each one no bigger than a toolshed, screen doors flapping half-unhinged in the sticky summer afternoon. A gaggle of children with mussed black hair are playing with toys in the dirt. A brown girl chases a taller brown boy, squealing when he waves a rubber dolly barely out of her reach.

Long grey metal buildings with oversized garage doors must be machine sheds or shops. Monstrous battered tractors are parked willy-nilly, engine parts scattered on the ground. Joy may not know a caterpillar from a skid steer, but she does know her father took better care of his machinery than this guy. Alongside mounds of tree bark and shavings are heaps of firewood cut into stove lengths. A brindle-coloured mongrel rushes out, teeth bared, barks at the tires, then jumps up, his claws scratching the green paint on the Merc. Joy leans on the horn. It's a good thing she left Jemima back at the cabin.

A man in grimy blue jeans and no shirt emerges from one of the buildings and hollers at the dog. "Rufus, scarper!" He lifts one boot off the ground and Rufus vamooses, his tail between his legs. Joy steps out and states her name in a no-nonsense tone to the man, presumably McPherson. High-pitched squeals of an electric saw, like a dentist's drill, make her head ache. He semaphores to another man to throw wood into Joy's trailer. Then he stands in one spot, an inch of roll-your-own pinched in the corner of his mouth, and concentrates on Joy. "What's a bonnie lass like you doin' haulin' her own firewood?" She chooses not to answer. His chest is the colour of the sand on Cavendish Beach. Above a rearing stallion on his belt buckle, moist copper hairs curlicue playfully around his bellybutton and further up around his nipples. He hikes up his pants and rests one calloused hand on Joy's dented trailer. His middle finger is missing. "You know this half-cord won't see you through the winter. It's gauna be a cauld'un and a lang'un."

"I know," she replies, even though she doesn't.

He pushes back his Husqvarna cap, wipes his forehead with a rag, and takes Joy's cheque. Sweat drips from his dark armpit hair. The muscles in his shoulders shift. He stinks of fuel oil.

As Joy eases her foot off the brake and onto the gas pedal, she hears through the open window, "Whare sits our sulky, sullen dame . . ." Of all the goddam nerve!

Wending her way back along the soft road, she keeps one eye on her rear-view mirror to make sure the trailer hasn't come unhitched. Earl never showed her how to fasten the safety chain.

Does McPherson pay his men minimum wage? The man who loaded her wood had not uttered one word. Strong back, weak mind, no sass, no talk of a labour union.

Ruminating over the scene at the Crossing, Joy unloads the trailer and piles the wood on the deck close to the door. Should she report that son-of-a-bitch to the Department of Labour or mind her own business? At least those men have jobs and aren't on social assistance.

In the cabin, she practises the violin, easily ignoring dust bunnies under the furniture and cat hair on the kitchen table. In a sing-song voice, her mother used to say (about a neighbour), "She sure isn't much of a housekeeper." Neither is Joy, but when was there time with teaching plus working Saturdays and summer holidays at the drycleaners to pay off Earl's debts? Besides, cleaning the house was futile with three boys missing the toilet.

Early August is blueberry season, clusters of frosty blue in contrast with grey-green moss, yellowing pine needles, and botany beige sand. One ice cream pailful should last the winter. Tomorrow morning, she will be stiff from bending over. Tonight, her supper will be a blueberry sundae in a soup bowl.

With a foreboding chill in the evening air, Joy cannot put off a second trip to the sawmill any longer. She doesn't bother phoning ahead this time. McPherson and two of his men are bent over a tractor with its guts exposed. High-pitched squealing comes from a welding torch, sparks flying, on the far side of the yard. The men, probably from Wapiskaw Mahihkan Reserve, leave the tractor and begin loading the trailer. "Hist it up," McPherson snarls. "We gotta get this bastard up and rinnin' today." This time, Joy hands her cheque to one of the men, his mouth hanging open, expressionless.

Can they leave on their days off? Where is there to go? Digger's for a hamburger, fries, and a Pepsi? Bicycles lie in the weeds alongside rusted shells of stripped cars with their hoods up. Why aren't there any women in sight? How do they endure the engines roaring, screams of saws, men shouting, wood banging against wood, the pings of metal, the din of industry? And the smell of diesel. Joy has been mouth-breathing since she got out of her car.

McPherson is turning a wrench on the tractor, a greasy rag hanging from his waist. A little girl in pink shorts sidles up to him. He stops what he's doing, reaches into a pocket at her eye level, and pulls out a roll of Life Savers. He separates a green one with his thumbnail and hands it to her. "Here you go, Tottie." She pops it into her mouth. Then he gives her a white one. "For your sister, too." The autumn sun highlights gold strands in the unruly red hair poking out of his sweat-stained cap.

Joy dodges beer bottles and tin cans, and navigates the Merc out of the yard, with Rufus nipping at the tires. In the distance is a two-storey log house with dormer windows, a fieldstone chimney, and a wraparound porch.

Back home, she unhitches the trailer, but can't face the task of carrying and stacking more wood. Men, either they're namby-pamby or there's testosterone oozing from their pores, she thinks, remembering a T-shirt she wore in the seventies, with the slogan: "A woman needs a man like a fish needs a bicycle."

Poplars cast a strong scent in the golden month of October. Joy lies on the ground to take in the last of the rustling leaves. Buds have formed, waiting to burst open in spring and paint the trees with dabs of green. What a damn fool she has been all these years believing buds are a sign of spring. Has she told the boys she wants to be buried under a poplar tree, not next to Earl in that stark cemetery with tombstones on a grid, and a map at the entrance? Looking up through yellow leaves to blue sky, she hums a line from Connie Kaldor: *You can hear it in the rustle of the poplar leaves at the bend in the river they call Batoche.* Eyes closed, she pretends it's the sound of the ocean, imagines McPherson's heft.

Her reading glasses rest on the cover of *Small Wonder*. She feels a pang of loneliness. A winter without human company, indoor plumbing, TV, or the Internet will be tough. She will find out if the lake gradually forms a solid mass, or begins freezing from the shoreline and works its way out. Will chunks of ice come and go with the wind until there is nowhere for them to move?

It comes in the night. Winter. Creeps in and lays a white blanket over the landscape while Joy is sleeping. If she'd known, she would have slept outside in a sleeping bag and awakened covered with snow like a homeless person under a city overpass. On spruce boughs, on prickly rose bushes, blueberry plants, the moss, and every skinny birch twig is a dusting of icing sugar. Neither human nor animal has yet disturbed it. Grey sky. It's a black-and-white photograph of a winter wonderland framed by her kitchen window, a scene from *Dr. Zhivago*.

To Joy, it feels like Christmas morning. What she wouldn't give for a wood-slat box filled with Jap oranges wrapped in green paper. Snow equals Christmas — hanging silver tinsel on a real tree, John Denver singing *Merry Christmas Little Zachary*, wrapping presents, making Nanaimo bars. None of the preparations can begin in earnest until her piece of earth is white.

Minus 6 degrees Celsius. Thank you Pierre Trudeau for the metric system. The condensation on the inside of the single-pane windows will freeze, a palette for Jack Frost to paint feathers. When Ross brings the children at Christmastime, they'll lie in bed, their warm breath on the windowpanes, scratching their own imaginative designs in the hoarfrost, just wait and see. Those energy-efficient windows have practically put Jack Frost out of business.

"Well Jemima, my girl, our footprints will be the first to mar the fresh snow." Joy pulls on her Sorel boots, mitts, and a toque, with the dog twirling at her feet in anticipation. They break trail across the yard and driveway, but further along on the road to the beach, there are fresh tracks of whitetail deer. Then come six-inch wide stretches dragged long and flat, and claw prints the size of a loonie. A beaver? A raccoon? The next time she's in the city, she'll have to stop at Chapters and look for a guide to wild animal tracks. The quiet of the snow speaks to her. The only sound is her breathing.

A demarcation between dark open water and white snow stuck onto ice is visible from shore. Joy bathes her face in rays of sun breaking through the bare poplar branches, and hums *Jesus Wants Me for a Sunbeam*, a tune from her Sunday School days at the Belle Oak Baptist Church. Rosy cheeks feel sooo good.

Where are those children from the Crossing? The sawmill must be a seasonal operation. Surely the families have relocated to houses with central heating, and the children are in school.

Ah, the elusive white-throated sparrow. She has seldom seen it, but knows its song. Four pensive whistles the same pitch, then three quavering notes. Her spirit bird . . . it followed her from the farm to the city and then faithfully to Otter Lake.

Tonight she will try to find Orion's belt. Her join-the-dots astronomy guide shows it in the northern hemisphere in winter. She studies the drawing, then goes out with Jemima at her heels. There it is, three bright stars in a row, the hunter's belt with the sword hanging down. It has been in the sky her entire life. The pitch darkness makes her quiver, a reminder that time has elapsed.

A Jarvis family lived on the same municipal road as Joy's family. Orion and Orpheus were their children's names. They were called *Or-yan* and *Or-fis*. During harvest, when Joy's father was busy combining wheat, she had to catch a ride to school with them. Their car was dirty and they all smelled of B.O. Mr. Jarvis, who worked at a warehouse, whistled with his arm poking out of the open car window. Some days he sang in a robust voice, the same song over and over.

Mickey Maloney ducked his head
when a bucket of whiskey flew at him.
Cryin will ye walup each girl and boy,
t-underin Jaysus, do ye think I'm dead?

Joy was mortified. She would mouth-breathe and stare out of her closed window until she exited the rust-eaten jalopy in front of the school.

Most of Joy's Christmas cards have been forwarded by the couple who bought her house. She declines Billy's invitation to spend Christmas at his place. AJ and Ross, with his wife and three children, come on Boxing Day for two nights. She wishes she could keep the little ones until after New Year's, when school reconvenes.

On Valentine's Day, she misses the flowers AJ has sent every year since his first job packing groceries. Sweet-natured AJ, caressing the shiny red paint on the Cutlass convertible, one of Earl's ill-conceived surprises. The three boys were in the driveway in bare feet when she arrived home from school, Ross in the driver's seat, and Billy asking Earl, "Did you really buy it for Mom?" The scenes were all much the same, Joy hitting the roof, Earl devastated, and the boys scattering to the furthest corners of the house, Earl pacing or operating power tools in the basement day and night, then crashing, sleeping from Friday after work straight through to Sunday suppertime. When he awoke, he would sidle up to her from the rear, arms around her waist, his hands wandering up to caress her breasts. "You wouldn't be giving your old man the silent treatment, would you?" Tuning out pleas from the boys, Joy would return Earl's latest purchase. "It'll be okay, Mom," AJ whispered. The flashback contains every detail of the scene, even the smell of Pizza Pops on AJ's breath.

The letter from Dr. Bhalla absolved Earl of responsibility for the purchases he made during a manic phase. "My husband isn't well," she said, and handed the letter and the car keys to the salesman, refusing to honour the credit card debit. After Earl's death, the psychiatrist reassured her there was nothing she could have done to prevent the suicide. Earl was in a depressive phase, he explained, and lab results confirmed he had not been taking his Lithium. *Pompous* was the word that came to Joy sitting across the desk from him.

We let the boys down, Earl and I, that's what Joy is thinking. At the funeral, the minister avoided the word "suicide". "Bad things sometimes happen to good people," he said. "Earl couldn't be the father his sons needed." Why did he say that? He had never even met Earl. Wasn't it enough that she requested donations to the CMHA in lieu of flowers? Earl was neither a hero nor a victim. He refused his injections because it impeded his sexual performance. One time, she found him huddled on the floor in the corner of the bedroom, whimpering. It was she who had been long-suffering and she who bore the wounds.

The year she went to Summer School in Saskatoon to finish up her BEd, she played with a study partner named Neil. They French-kissed and she let him unbutton her blouse, but when his fingers inched their way down her firm midriff and into her panties, she pulled away. After all, she was newly married and the church pianist.

Years later, after Earl's mental problems had taken hold, Joy considered taking the boys and leaving, but what if Earl killed himself?

It was a Wednesday after school. Earl's car was parked in the driveway. He must have left work early. Joy was greeted at the back door by Jemima and the girls. She placed her shoes on the mat beside Earl's, and started supper. There was a niggling in the pit of her stomach. "Earl?" She couldn't hear the radio in the bedroom. Sometimes he would lie on the bed and listen to FM before supper.

Lightheaded, swallowing, she called, "Earl?" Water boiling in a saucepan, ready for potatoes, a teaspoon of oil sizzling in the frying pan, she looked into the living room, walked down the hallway to the bedroom, the bathroom, the boys' bedrooms. She went down into the basement, stopped cold partway down the stairs. Earl was hanging from a beam beside the washer and dryer.

With her index finger, she brushes snow off the rusty pump handle, fills six four-gallon containers, and brings them into the cabin. One is needed beside the kitchen sink, another beside the toilet. She fills the Dutch oven and the canning kettle, brings them to a boil on the propane stove, empties them into the bathtub, then adds cold. All this effort for a measly three inches of warm water. At first, she did it every day, but her back and shoulders ached from carrying those pails, and her fingers were numb, so her bath has become a Saturday extravagance. In the city, soaking in a tub filled to the brim had been a must every evening. At least she can say she is managing without running water.

On bright white afternoons, she snowshoes across the lake, leans against a balsam fir, and drinks tea from a thermos. Monotonous frigid days blend into one, an interminable winter of her discontent, a psychological blizzard. Bored and leaden at times, unable to concentrate or focus, she stuffs herself with sweets and Christmas chocolates. Agitated at other times, she chews her cuticles, flits from one activity to another. Her mother would say she's at sixes and sevens. There's a name for this — cabin fever. Or is it melancholia? Whatever it's called, Joy is losing her connection. An early bedtime proves to be her salvation. Like Gran Sullivan, she gets up with the shickens and goes to bed with the shickens.

The ghetto at McPherson's Crossing feeds her disgruntlement, shelters cobbled together with salvaged lumber, tin, and cardboard dragged home from nuisance grounds. Even Indian reserves with third world standards, have real houses and swings for children. She has seen them for herself. Earl used to say she had a heart as big as a hotel. On the first day of school, she ached for children who couldn't write a paragraph about a summer road trip. She would slip a new red crayon into their boxes of used Crayolas because red was certain to be the missing colour. To her, the Crossing is a microcosm of social injustice, and burning McPherson's firewood makes her complicit.

In April, the temperature goes up and down like a whore's pants. The ice cries and growls as it softens. Will it go out and never come back? At the beach, will it melt gradually or will the shoreline resist? Boat docks can buckle and be dragged across the lake, she knows, shattered into pieces against the far shore. As the ice rots from underneath, it will turn black beneath its whiteness. Will it break from the banks of the creek and race downstream?

It is during an afternoon of violin practice that the stench of cat pee burns Joy's nostrils. She opens the windows on the sunny west side to allow in fresh air. On the six o'clock news, as Paul Martin offers lame excuses for the sponsorship scandal, she remembers riding her two-wheeler around the farmyard, dreaming of becoming the first female Prime Minister of Canada. She'd have done a hell of a lot better job than Paul Martin with his goofy grin.

Mother Nature refuses to fast-forward spring to meet one person's needs. Joy thrashes from one side of the double bed to the other. After a full year of sleeping alone, she can settle neither on her own side nor on Earl's. Restless ice, creaking and groaning as if it were alive, at long last lulls her to sleep. She twitches, fidgets, sleeps, kicks her legs, dreams, and repeatedly flips her pillow over, until a mysterious word rouses her. Eyes wide awake, her memory flashes back to a Clydesdale horse snagged on a strand of barbed wire concealed by tall grass. As she gropes her way to the bathroom in the dark, her father in striped overalls is leading his beloved Rex into the barn and tenderly cleansing his flank, then painting it with Lugol's iodine. Blood will rush in to heal the wound, he reassures Joy. It's nature's healing process. Moist, red bumps will form, then gradually dry out, and by fall a dark granular scar will take shape. Proudflesh, he calls the permanent scar. Proudflesh is stronger than healthy, untested skin.

No point in going back to bed. In the La-z-Boy, knees to chin, she envelopes herself like a chrysalis in the patchwork quilt her mother made for their wedding present. She doesn't think to stoke the fire to quell her shivers. Earl used to rub her frosty back in bed. "C'mere, I'll warm you up. I swear you must have been a cat in a previous life," he'd say. They hadn't made love the last two years. He couldn't. Ever since she was widowed, she never felt toasty warm at night. When was the last time a man had touched her? Oh yes, Ross had given her a perfunctory goodbye hug the last time she had been in town, and told her to drive safe.

Dawn breaks, and in the cozy haven of the woollen quilt, she imagines a man's clumsy hands stroking her more-than-enough breasts and soft belly, taking an interest in what lies between her dimply thighs. Is it too late for all that? For a' that and a' that.

It might do her good to get out, she thinks, but Digger's is the only gathering place within ninety miles, and the locals aren't her kind of people. The men talk about moose hunting or fishing for lake trout before the blight of summer weekenders. The few women look like men, short hair, lumberjack shirts, *tough broads*, Earl would call them, rough and ready, hardy-har-harring at every crude joke, toothless beyond the incisors, probably never read a book. But Digger's is the social hub in Joy's corner of the world. She swallows her pride, gives herself a proverbial kick in the ass, leaves the quilt in a heap on the chair, and makes porridge. A conversation and a taste of the real world, in contrast with left-wing CBC Radio, are her modest expectations of the 9:30 coffee klatch at Digger's. At least she'll have something fresh to think about.

The Merc weaves around potholes and broken asphalt. What if they're all guys? She'll just get her milk and newspaper, and exit. Muddy, salt-encrusted 4 x 4 trucks are filed parallel in the parking lot, some with big dogs pacing in the box. The sign reads: "DIGGER'S — Outfitter, Store, Café, Cabin + Boat Rentals, STC Bus Depot". In the porch is a stack of empty plastic Mazola Oil pails. "$1.00 each. 2/$1.50. Make great water pales". She stomps the slush off her sneakers, takes a deep breath, and walks into the dimly lit store. A rotary rack has *Betty and Veronica* comics, *ATV Trail Rider, Playboy, Guns and Ammo.* In behind is a sloping display of chocolate bars, Life Savers, Cheezies, and Sen-Sen. Along the wall on home-made shelves are basic groceries — Heinz Beans with Pork, Chuckwagon Stew, Carnation Evaporated Milk, Jiffy popcorn in foil pie plates, along with tarps and Spic 'n Span. Fishing lures and mousetraps are hanging on pegboard.

At the one long table, the chatter is about a priest who caught an eighteen-pound walleye. One of the men repeats what he read in *The Nipawin Journal:* "He says he got the nibble in an ice-fishing shack at Tobin Lake. Praying and jigging." Guffaws. Through cigarette smoke, the talk comes around to spring break-up, the Lotto 649, tabloid news, the price of gas, and back to spring break-up. Joy pours herself a coffee, "Self-Serve. $1.00. Free refills", and takes a seat at the table. If they notice her arrival, they give no indication, which is a relief. Do they know about Earl's suicide? Maybe it was the topic of conversation a year ago when the gossip first reached here via moccasin telegraph.

An old man, a dumpling with pink droopy earlobes and a grey fringe of clipped hair, works himself into a lather. "The Arthur-itis Brothers paid me a visit. I'm so stiff I can hardly get up off the shitter." When he lets out a donkey laugh, folds of skin reduce his eyes to slits. His tongue darts in and out. One fella hoots, slaps his knee, and contributes his own testimonial to aging. With a marked politeness, Joy listens to the twittering group, but her attention is drawn toward T-shirts hanging in her line of vision. White or baby blue T-shirts with factory-emblazoned fish writhing at the end of fishing lines, or black bears posing against a backdrop of evergreens. Take your pick, a fish or a bear adorned with an iron-on decal, "Digger's, Otter Lake, SASK" in Gothic font. On chairs pushed back from the table, big-bellied men with an assortment of facial hair and soiled hunting caps (some fluorescent), snort and gurgle. They look like boozers, she thinks, red-faced, ripe for a heart attack.

Spring break-up is a big deal. A beaky woman with a liver-spotted face is one of the boys. Her mouth drops open, exposing a plug of chewing tobacco. "Just wait till that water pressure builds up on the lake. Mark my words, there'll be an explosion." The way she thrusts her head forward reminds Joy of a goose crossing the barnyard. "I been watchin' it every spring for fourteen years now. It's gonna snap. But it's not warm enough yet." This advance information is of use to Joy once she gets past the woman's protruding mottled brown teeth. If Earl were here, he would've made eye contact with Joy, then the knuckle of his index finger would've pushed up the tip of his nose. Toffee-nose.

By 10:30, the crowd is thinning. Joy pays no attention to bruised apples and wilted heads of lettuce, but reaches into a freezer and takes out a cardboard container of whole milk jammed in alongside wieners, white Wonder Bread, and Fudgsicles furry with frost. It will take twelve hours at room temperature for the milk to thaw. Next to the cash register, on rusted white metal shelving, are Band-Aid Tough-Strips, Rolaids, and Extra-Strength Tylenol. Jack knives, lottery tickets, and men's Timex watches are secure under glass.

On the counter is a sheet of cardboard divided into squares like a Grey Cup pool, with "SPRING BREAK-UP" printed in black felt marker. To lay a bet, you leave a toonie in the envelope and write your name in the square along with your prediction of the day spring break-up will happen. Might there be a dispute over the precise definition of "spring break-up", Joy wonders. Do all of the chunks of ice have to be set in motion, or will evidence of open water be sufficient? That argument must have been settled years earlier with the original Spring Break-Up Pool. Who will be the judge?

"Milk, the newspaper, and a coffee," she says to Digger.

"Four twenty-five," he barks.

Without warning, blood rushes to Joy's head, and her heart begins to pound in her ears. Instinctively, she can sense McPherson close behind her. Hot breath sets fire to her neck and a lusty brogue fans the flames. "I haird tremblin' violin strings playin' *Bonny Jean of Aberdeen* . . ." A bristle of copper moustache, flecked with silver, and strong smiling teeth affront her when she reels around. " . . . when I drove by your playce, that is." His look is penetrating. The moist red expanse of his mouth is edged by wind-chapped lips. A droplet of spit tickles a crack in his lower lip. His nostrils flare like the wild stallion on his belt buckle. He presses his bulk closer. The brush of heavy flannel gives rise to pinpricks in Joy's fingers gripping the milk and newspaper close to her chest. She turns to pay Digger. Tongue-tied, she walks out. She has to get some air. Did McPherson purposely blow on the nape of her neck? Cocky bastard! Last night's whiskey on his breath.

Foul Play Not Suspected

BUN DOUGH RISING AND SPILLING OVER the top of a mixing bowl. White dough where my waist used to be. Zigzagged with silver grooves, spattered with purple. My breasts are empty sacks flattened by a rolling pin, puckered pinkish-brown nipples circled by niplets. The scar from my hysterectomy is dark and crumpled like last year's rhubarb under melting April snow. Sitting on the toilet mustering the energy to wipe my backside, there's ample time to survey my nether regions. I'm hacking thanks to thirty years of Earl's cigarette smoke. It's a dry cough, as we say on the prairies.

I'm sniffling as usual. Earl used to say he could tell my where-abouts by the sound of me sniffling. Come to think of it, Earl always liked to know where I was, period. He had a jealous streak. I blow my nose first thing every morning, like a farmer. For the rest of the day, I sniffle. There's no one to be bothered by it any more.

I've gotten into the habit of wiping myself from the front. I'll pull my underpants up to my knees, make sure the Kotex pad is in place. Honestly, I drip like a leaky tap. Surely one of the boys will tell me if I start to smell of urine. Heave-Ho! I'm standing.

Steady now, pull my panties up the rest of the way. Now I have to turn around, put the lid down, and flush. What brain surgeon decided the handle belongs there? All this effort just to take a morning poop! My coffee should be ready by now.

The room's spinning. What am I doing on top of the toilet lid? I must've passed out. Geez, I have to pee so bad I can't hold it. Is this another one of those weak spells? It feels different, though. Damn it, I can't lift my arm or move my hand. And this leg's asleep.

The sun is in the western sky, so it must be evening. Last thing I remember, it was morning. Bathrooms need fresh air and a window. The houses in that expensive new subdivision just have ceiling fans in the bathrooms, Ross said. Where would I keep my cold cream and my denture cup if I didn't have a window ledge? Paint's peeling, putty's brittle.

The phone. That'll be AJ. He'll think I'm out in the garden fussing with my daylilies. Look at the mess I've made. The bathroom's flooded. Better take off this wet underwear before I get a chill. It's hard with one arm. Please God . . . not a stroke.

Jemima, you can squeeze through, can't you? That's my girl. You don't understand. It's okay if you piddle in the house. I did.

I should be able to figure this out. It's Wednesday, AJ works nights, he won't call again till Friday after he's slept. I'm in trouble. I have to get to the phone. I'll hang onto the towel rack and slide down off the seat. Easy does it.

Ah, the dawn chorus. Mourning doves, crows, the distant hum of traffic on the highway. This oilcloth is like ice. When I was a little girl, I loved to skate and I was good at it, too. I'd fall down on the ice and get right up again a hundred times, no problem. My arm's bleeding a little. Bubbly veins, onionskin, dirt under my stubby nails from pulling the first carrots of the season. That was the last thing I ate.

These teary eyes, I keep a box of Kleenex in every room. No use even trying to read first thing in the morning, I have to keep lifting my bifocals to blot my eyes. It's like I saved up all my tears, didn't shed 'em, though God knows I had plenty of reasons.

If I lived in that Pioneer Manor, there'd be an emergency pull cord right beside the toilet, I bet, just like in the hospital. But the name of the place is enough to put a person off. *Pioneer.* My Gran was a pioneer for Chrissake, not me. Ross has been dropping hints. "Just think, Mom, wouldn't it be nice if you didn't have to bother cooking?" Here in my own place I can eat Cream of Wheat for supper if I feel like it, scuffle around in my slippers, leave things in a mess, and it's nobody's business.

How in Hell am I going to get out of here? These legs served me well till now, could've given Marco Polo a run for his money. Now they're next to useless. My thighs aren't even dimpled anymore, just loose skin and purple veiny patches. I always dreaded bathing suits.

This oilcloth takes me back to summer holidays with Gran and Grandad. It's cracking at the seams where somebody nailed it down. AJ painted the walls turquoise, like I asked him, to match the diamonds on the red background. He made a snide remark about the bare light bulb, but I left it anyway, string hanging.

I must be quite a sight half naked, wedged between the toilet and the door. Gaunt arse and shrivelled tits. Earl never paid any attention to them, used to say, "I grabbed onto enougha those milking cows on the farm." But Scotty . . . that was another story.

I'd be making us a cup of tea and he'd undo my buttons from behind. He'd take off my shirt, then my brassiere, and I'd wriggle my titties till they danced. He'd chase me to the bedroom in the cabin, slapping my bum. Then he'd get down on his knees like he was about to propose. He'd cup one breast in each hand and make love to them each in turn. I'd watch his eyelashes flicker, the tip of his tongue going round and round my hard nipples, teasing me, my fingers kneading his scalp, tugging on that thick head of copper hair. It makes my crotch tighten up remembering it.

My tongue darts in and out in search of the next word when I'm talking. From the corners of my mouth, furrows lead down to my chin like riverbeds, and in them drool floweth. With a crumpled serviette, I dabbeth.

I'm outta practice, but here goes. God in heaven . . . I sound funny without my top plate in. Is this how it's going to end for me? Stuck in the bathroom? Better than getting shot in a war or killed in a car crash, I suppose. Or cancer, that's what I'm scared of, a long drawn-out affair. Thank you for my sons, they've been the light in my life. And thank you for the times I forgot my troubles and laughed out loud. For my flower garden, Oh Henry chocolate bars, that trip to the Maritimes. Funny, when I boil it all down, I didn't expect that much out of life. I'm proud of myself for teaching school, helping out some old folks in my spare time. But you know all that. Forgive me for the times I hurt anybody. I must've hurt Earl, being so hostile after his manic spells. And the boys, they were hurt when I moved up north, so far away from my grandchildren.

But how could I stay in that house? Every time I went down into that basement, I saw Earl hanging from a beam beside the washer and dryer, the laundry basket full of clean socks, his socks waiting to be sorted into matching pairs. *In sickness and in health till death do us part.* Now I live with the guilt. It keeps me company every waking hour.

And there was that messy business with Ralph, but Betty jumped to her own conclusions. She never liked me anyway.

Never could figure out why Gran and Grandad left this place. All of a sudden. Mother said there'd been a bit of bother, whatever that means.

How long can a body go without food or water? It's been a couple of days. There's scum on my tongue. I'll try to pull myself up off the floor, get a drink from the tub. This porcelain's even colder than the linoleum. Now if I can just get my elbow onto the edge. Damn, I can't reach the tap, not even that one droplet dangling from the faucet. I'm parched. I'll slid back down. Ouch, my whole side's gonna be bruised.

Maybe Lucy will notice there are no lights coming on or off, and send someone to check on me. She'd be able to see that from her trailer. I was going to give her a call after I got settled in, but the boys said, "Don't even think about it Mother. She's crazy, took a pot-shot at the sheriff. Keep your distance." Too bad, we used to be playmates. Haven't seen her since we were ten years old. Heard she's had a hard time of it. I always see her drive by in that beat-up van.

I'm starting to fidget and twitch like the old ladies in the nursing home. Tapping my fingers on my withered thigh. Mother's head used to jerk to the side and one of her shoulders would shrug for no reason. She'd rub the pilly fabric of her skirt, roll up the edge, then unroll it, roll it up again, unroll it.

Olga died on the toilet. Had that awful flu bug, diarrhea and vomiting at the same time, choked on her vomit, sitting on the toilet. The least her kids could've done was make up a different story. "Did you hear about Olga? Died on the toilet, poor dear." That's how she'll be remembered, not for bringing up two grandchildren when that hare-brained Bobbi-Sue took off with a new boyfriend. I suppose I'll be remembered for dying on the bathroom floor.

It can't be more than ten degrees in here. Sure cools off at night. If only I could reach the window and knock down the stick that's propping it open.

I'm sorry, Jemima Puddleduck, you can't figure out why I'm not in my chair, can you? There should be enough food and water in your bowls. Here, cuddle up beside me. Good puppy. Keep me warm.

I really believed I'd live to see ninety like Gran. Even told the boys they should expect me to be a burden. Instead, I'm dying by inches on this bathroom floor and AJ will be the one to find me. I'll be cold and stiff. It'll break his heart.

So what am I going to miss out on? Adult diapers, books on tape read by some Hollywood actress, getting ripped off by a hearing aid salesman, my appetite gone the way of taste and smell, pills set out on the kitchen table one week at a time by a cheery little Home Care nurse, being forced to move into that Pioneer Manor . . . now there's a good reason to breathe my last breath right here in my own bathroom.

I've grown kinda fond of this bellyfat, like a child worrying a blanket. It's what they call *an apron of fat*. Seems to me the funeral home must embalm a lot of aprons, all of us church ladies who baked too many date squares for our own good.

Wait just a minute God. That is, if you're paying attention to what's going on down here. I've got a few more things to get off my chest.

How come I couldn't have a diamond ring on my twenty-fifth anniversary, like Betty? Every time there was a little extra cash, Earl would blow it on some damn fool thing, like that red Cutlass convertible. He could be such an impulsive bugger. Would a kind-hearted husband, a set of wedding rings, and some decent furniture have been too much to ask for? I've been thinking about buying a new couch. Mine's been covered up with an afghan for so long I can barely remember what colour it is. Ah you've got more important things to do than listen to an old woman complain. Like stopping the bloodbath in Iraq. I'll say Amen, and please send an angel to watch over my boys and their little ones.

Oh, I suppose I better add the wives, too.

I have to dig deep. This is my last chance. I had sex with two men and only one of them was my husband. In high school, I necked with a few boys in the back seat and, at university, Greg and I played touchy-feely but were scared to go all the way. My conscience is clear in the sex department.

Did I do anything I'm ashamed of? I should've left Earl, that's my biggest regret. He made all of us crazy. We never knew what was coming next. My own sister got divorced, but oh no! not Goody-Two-Shoes Joy, she took her marriage vows before God and a churchful of witnesses and she kept her promise.

It's time to cut through the bullshit. Tell the truth. God, you know it already, so I just have to tell it to myself. Out loud. I've thought it, but I've never said it out loud. What happened that morning before school when Ross and AJ were fighting over the toaster and Earl grabbed both of them by one ear . . . it was ugly. I had to step in before he knocked them senseless. I kept Ross home for a couple of days because his earlobe was torn, should've taken him to the hospital to have it stitched. Told him his Dad was under a lot of stress at work. Rented Nintendo games. Sent him back to school with a sick note.

I never slept with Earl again. I remembered *Lysistrata* from English 101. Moved his clothes down to the basement, put his underwear and socks into a musty-smelling chiffonier that used to be his parents'. There weren't even partitions, just an old bunk bed on a frayed remnant of carpet in a corner. Not far from the washing machine, come to think of it. He curtained it off, suspended a piece of pipe between two teleposts to hang up his shirts and pants, and slept there for the last three years of his life. I refused to change his sheets or vacuum. I was cold as a fish, believed I was standing up for the boys.

What I should've done the day of the toaster episode was get the hell out. I could've rented a house. How many times have I gone over it? Marriage vows. Keeping the family together. It's a lie. I've been telling myself a real doozy all these years. The truth is I was afraid of looking like a failure. It was pride. That's what it was. Pride's one of the seven deadly sins, isn't it? On my deathbed, it comes to me like a revelation. My own personal *Book of Revelation*.

I should've gone to church more often, but when you pray for your husband to take his prescriptions and he won't, it's hard to sit in a pew singing, "*What a friend we have in Jesus take it to the Lord in prayer.*" Come to think of it, I haven't set foot in a church since Earl's funeral. I could've sent more money to those poor AIDS orphans in Africa instead of buying some cockamamie gadget advertised on TV. But if you think I deserve to go to heaven anyway, I'd sure like to put my arms around my Gran one more time. I never had a chance to tell her she was my hero. Amen.

Good timing, eh Jemima? I just said my prayers, it's dark, now I lay me down to sleep.

I can't keep still. Just like in bed, except it's usually both legs jumping around. My blankets are always in a jumble by morning. A chill must turn into pneumonia eventually. That's what this is . . . eventually. There'll be an autopsy to determine the cause of my death. A person can't just die of old age anymore. "Joy Werner died of natural causes," that's what they'll type on some government form. "Foul play not suspected." Surely the police won't have to get involved.

In a way, the bathroom's a fitting place to die. One minute your body's working, the next minute it stops, you mess yourself, then rigor mortis sets in.

C'mere Jemima Puddleduck, you're a good girlie. Keep your old pal company, will you? AJ will take you home.

Jesus loves me, this I know.

A Bit of Bother

AT THE INTERSECTION, AN ARROW POINTS the way to Devil's Beach. Someone painted the two words on a board from a picket fence and nailed it to the signpost, below "Yield". The sign has slipped and the arrow is, in fact, pointing downward at an angle toward the gravel road. Lucy turns at the corner. She is on her way to the beach. It's only eleven o'clock, so no one will be there yet. The day promises to be a scorcher.

She parks, opens the door, pulls the lever to engage the hydraulic lift, wheels herself onto the mesh platform, and lowers it to ground level. She slides out of the wheelchair with her sweat-pants still on, bathing suit underneath, and pushes herself across the sand with both elbows like a cross-country skier working her poles. It's a good thing she hasn't put on any weight. The sun burns her bare shoulders. Close to the shoreline, she wriggles from side to side tugging at her pants, leaving them behind. She keeps her elbows going until she is in the water, then dogpaddles out a ways and does a dead man's float. The cool lake water soothes her flushed face, her oily complexion, her pimples. She flips over onto her back and lets the current carry her out, but not too far. Back to front, front to back, five minutes or so on each side, then she paddles back to shore. The crawl to the van is gruelling. She repeats the steps in reverse order until she's back in the driver's seat, takes off the top half of her bathing suit and changes into a T-shirt. No one will notice her wet crotch.

In Redbird, she stops at the post office to pick up her mail, then at the Co-op for bread, a jar of Cheez Whiz, and a carton of Marlboros. She parks in the lot behind the Belly-Up Bar and smushes her cigarette in the ashtray. Once she's lowered her chair onto the ground, she aims for the Offsale door. It's Friday afternoon, they'll be expecting her.

" . . . when you're stokin' the fire." Lucy catches the tail-end of the punchline, followed by a burst of laughter. It's a send-off, a round of drinks for Reiny Pfeifer who is leaving the farm for a job in Regina, third generation on that section of land, can't make a go of it. The waitress brings her a Pil.

"Last one to go was Burkardt," someone says.

"Nah, Jamiesons were after him."

"How about Bill Friesen?"

It's a roll-call, the names of single men and families who rented out their land and went to the city.

Lucy lights up, relishes the drag, then raises her jaw and blows the smoke up into the haze. "There's one person moved back here," she says. "Sullivans' granddaughter, Joy. I call her 'Toots'. Same age as me. Seven zero. She's fixing up that old house. It's like trying to make a silk purse out of a sow's ear, if you ask me." She drops her chin back into the folds of her neck. "I say she won't last the winter. If trampin' through the snow to feed that pet cow don't change her mind, I might have to change it for her. Bring me another brewski, would ya?" She's guzzling her third.

Rusnak tips up the brim of his blaze orange hunting cap and tells her to quit being such a bitch.

Bittner, with his hangdog expression, adds, "Joy Sullivan's had a rough go of it. Her husband hung himself, ya know. Three boys still at home when he done it."

"And what about *my* little brother?" Condensation from the beer glass drips onto Lucy's lap.

"Gawd, you're still holdin' a grudge after all these years? It wasn't Joy that killed him, it was her grandad. An' he never got over it."

"Tough shit!" Lucy flicks off the ash, then tucks the cigarette in her pants pocket and backs away from the table. "I'm outta here."

In her van, she lights the half-ciggie with a red Bic, sucks in a breath, and balances it on the ashtray. "Gotta do somethin' about these gears stickin'." She can't afford to trade in the rattle-trap. "C'mon." She ups the volume of her voice. "Into reverse, you piece o' crap."

On her way past the Sullivan place, she looks sideways. Just one bullet hole through a window might do it, she thinks. Toots' Merc is gone. She's probably in Redbird at her son's place for supper.

Lucy hasn't seen Joy Sullivan close up since they were little girls pretending to be fancy ladies. Under the carragana hedge draped with a worn bedspread, they'd put on Joy's Grandma's old nylon blouses and nighties. While Joy dressed the barn kittens in doll clothes, poking holes in the pants for their tails, Lucy turned to her Dinky toys. She pulled a miniature manure spreader around in the gravel with her Massey Harris tractor while Joy pushed the doll carriage with hobbled kittens climbing out and having to be tucked back in.

Mrs. Sullivan would bring out a tray with peanut butter sandwiches and pink lemonade in plastic glasses. "Here's a little lunch for you girls." Lucy wasn't invited into the house, not once. At suppertime, Mrs. Sullivan would say, "You run along home now." Lucy's mother told her Sullivans were high class.

Joy spent the summer holidays on her grandparents' farm. Her grandfather called her Toots, so Lucy did, too. Toots was cute with her big cow eyes, a prissy smile, and permed blonde hair. Lucy has always been mousy-looking. In school pictures, there she is with stringy brown hair cut short just like today, except now it's gray and even thinner. When she looks into the mirror low down over the bathroom sink, she can see her father's face. After his stroke that is, when the meat fell off his bones. He used to holler, "Turn me over," in the middle of the night and Lucy would stuff Kleenex in his pie hole so she could get some sleep before work. Just the other day, when she was bedding in new brake pads on the van, she vowed she heard him gripe. "Whaddya doin' that for? They're still good. Don't you know they'll scream at you when they're worn out?"

Lucy lives in a trailer on the farm where she was born and raised. The house in the next yard, the Sullivan place, was deserted for years until three months ago, when Toots moved in. Rusnak rents the land. Lucy saw the truck hauling in corrugated aluminum panels. The house sure looks different with a blue roof and blue trim around the doors and windows. Toots must've left the weather-beaten siding to make it look original. Her sons did a first-rate job of cleaning up the yard, with their young ones darting in and out between the granaries, chasing Toots' little white dog. They rototilled a garden plot and fenced in a pasture for her cow. Lucy watched the goings-on from her front window. Must be nice having kids who help out.

A cow, if that ain't stupid. It's got no shelter. It'll freeze to death.

Toots has picked at a scab by showing up here. What does she think she's doing? Unless maybe her mother left the home quarter to her. It's been sixty years since Old Man Sullivan killed Wassail, ran over him with the hay mower. Lucy can't make any sense of it.

If Lucy knew which of her neighbours had poisoned her watchdog, she'd fire a gunshot through his windshield without a moment's hesitation. She took a potshot at the sheriff who came to repossess one of her vehicles, to scare him off. She could've hit him, but knew better. She landed in the Psych Centre, transportation courtesy of a paddy wagon. "It should've been me under the haymower," that's what she told the doctor who admitted her.

She plunks her groceries on the counter, wheels into the living room, and makes a U-turn in the worn grooves in the shag carpet. Car magazines are strewn about. She pulls the chain dangling from a swag lamp that resembles an olive, and uses the remote to turn on the TV. Oprah appears, lips in motion. "Every human being wants to be heard. You. You are not alone." On one of Lucy's walls is a photo of a white '65 Shelby GT with two wide blue stripes starting at the trunk and making their way up over the roof.

Lucy is oblivious to the fug. She lights a cigarette. Ashes spill over the ashtray next to the Twilite Motel & Bar coffee mug on a TV table. Her sagging couch is covered with a plush *Happy Holidays* blanket, a Christmas present from Larry. Her favourite poster is black-and-white, Marilyn Monroe, all cleavage, lolling against a classic car while Elvis strums his guitar on the rear bumper. Only Marilyn's lipstick and the taillights are coloured red.

The first time Lucy's father let her sit behind the wheel of the Fargo pick-up, she put it in reverse and popped the clutch, practically put both of them through the windshield. His spittle, his garlic breath, and his string of curses in Ukrainian jolted her, but the driving lesson continued. By age fifteen, she could handle the Massey 36, work the summerfallow by herself.

Her first fixer-upper was a 1960 Chevy Corvair with a rear-mounted engine, five on the floor, and bucket seats. She painted the body with a four-inch brush. Her old man called the colour "baby-shit yellow". When the paint was still tacky, she test-drove it to Devil's Beach. It was a Saturday afternoon and two boys from her class were in the shallow water fighting over an inflated ball, showing off for their girlfriends suntanning on blankets.

The girls wiggled their little butts over to where Lucy had stopped, the boys tagging along like the tails of kites. The girl in a bikini (who would die of an overdose in grade eleven) gushed, "Nice jalopy, Lucy. Love the colour." One of the boys drilled the ball at Lucy's flat chest. "C'mon Luce, trow da ball." What could you expect with a name like Ukrainetz? The carcass of the yellow Corvair is along the fence line, wheels up on railroad ties, the radio and tail lights gone, the passenger door wired shut. It was the car she used for her driver's test the day she turned sixteen.

Before she got knocked up, Lucy rebuilt a two-tone '52 Ford Customline Club, powder blue on the bottom, white on top. After school and on weekends, she'd poke around under the hood, arse sticking out. It's in her line of vision from the bedroom window. Turkey foot grass has grown up around the bumpers. There are gopher holes under the rusted-out wheels. "Disgraced the family," that was what her father said when he picked up her and Baby Phyllis at the hospital and dropped them off at Chow's Café. She had one room with a hotplate and sink, toilet down an outside flight of stairs and in through the back door. The same bathroom customers used.

When Lucy had to move back to the farm to look after her father, Phyllis took off for Calgary, and Lucy buried herself in fixing up cars. The finished products are parked alongside the '52 Ford. The junkers were towed out back, a ways over from Wassail's bicycle.

The winter after the old man died, Lucy was coming home from the bar one night, goading the ski-doo way too hard. She hit an icy mound, veered to one side, missed the approach to the old railroad bridge, and piled into one of the concrete buttresses. All she can remember is muttering "Hail Mary". She landed in a snowbank, paralyzed from the waist down. It's coming up fifteen years. The mangled '71 Nordic is with the other wrecks.

Phyllis had the porch built while Lucy was in Rehab after her accident. It's a shelter from the elements, and muck and slush can drip from her wheels onto the plank floor. Phyllis also found a used van with hand controls. The insurance paid for it.

Oprah, the queen of daytime talk is blabbering with women who work in pink ghettoes, but Lucy isn't paying attention. She's still toying with the idea of putting a hole through Toots' window. Not to hurt her, just make her think twice about living by herself in that farmhouse. Lucy wheels to the kitchen, grabs two bottles of beer from the fridge door, uses one to crack the cap off the other, puts one back.

Being alone on Friday nights is nothing new. It's Wednesdays Lucy dreads. Wednesdays used to be hers and Larry's. He was her only serious boyfriend. The bullies in high school called her "Lucy Loose Hole" even though she wasn't easy. Larry was the first travelling salesman she ever met. He sold Windsor Salt. She was wearing a T-shirt with PMS in great big letters across the boobs the first time she waited on him at the bar, before she even knew his name. He read the fine print and hooted. "I'm not Putting Up with Men's Shit." They always said it was that T-shirt that brought them together.

Luce and Lare never went out in public, just stayed in Room 32 at the Twilite Motel. He used to fart in bed on purpose, push her head under the blankets and make her smell it. Called it "a Dutch oven". It was good for a laugh. Larry's wife was a sour-puss, so he was glad to be on the road from Monday to Friday. He'd walk across the hall to the Off-Sale counter for a case of beer, order a pizza, or pick up burgers and onion rings at the A & Dub on his expense account. They'd watch TV and talk about everything under the sun. He gave her Chanel Number 5 perfume, a pointy black diamond ring, that leather jacket hanging on the hook in the kitchen. It went on for a couple of years until the company changed his route.

Larry used to tell her she had a bum like a tame bee. He liked to do it doggy-style. "You must've won the trophy for the nicest ass at your graduation."

She said she never finished grade twelve.

"Well, you would've won."

She was a housekeeper at the motel, so she made sure the rooms on either side of theirs were empty on Wednesday nights.

Oprah says, "You have to stand up for yourself. If you don't, who will?" One minute, Lucy's picking at her cuticles with a jackknife in front of the TV, the familiar comfort of beer and tobacco on her tongue. Next minute, she's putting on her leather jacket and heading out the door.

She brakes in the mouth of Toots' driveway with a .22 behind the driver's seat. She hasn't been here since she was a kid riding a bike. After the Sullivans took the crop off that fall, they deserted the place and never came back. Lucy was ten years old when Wassail was killed, old enough to know it was her fault. She was supposed to be watching him.

Toots is not at home. Lucy turns the wheel to line up her side of the van with one of the windows in the house. Must be the kitchen. The bottom corner of a flimsy white curtain is being sucked outside by the warm breeze. Just one bullet hole should do it. She shifts into Park, leaves the engine running, cranks her window down halfway. Reaches back for the gun, then into the glove compartment for the ammo. Loads one bullet, rests the barrel on the top edge of the glass, sets the sight at the middle of the windowpane more or less. The sun draws her eyes momentarily to the liver spots on her trigger hand. Chin on the rest, she closes one eye, looks through the sight, pauses. She pulls the trigger, then leans back in her seat. She's pretty sure she hit the window. Better get the Hell out of here.

She sips on a beer, cuts a piece off a coil of *kubasa* sausage, and chops onions, all the while adding up what she's got to show for her seventy years of living. Not much to add. A car collection and a daughter who visits once a year. She takes out six store-bought *pryohy*, puts the rest back in the freezer. After she's dead, Phyllis will have to pay somebody to haul away the vehicles before the property can be put up for sale. No one will be interested in the farmstead regardless of the spruce shelterbelt. Her trailer, the old house, granaries, and barn will collapse into a heap, just like every other place between here and town.

Toots must be getting three pensions, maybe even four. Must be nice to be a widow. Lucy has to make her Old Age Pension cheque stretch to the end of the month, but she's used to being hard up. The payment from renting out the land barely covers the taxes. She fought with Canada Pension Plan for years after her accident. "I'm sick of filling out your Goddam forms. Keep your money you cocksuckers!" That's exactly what she wrote on the back of one of their letters.

With a long-handled metal spoon, Lucy drops one frozen *pryohy*, then another into a pot on the stove. Waits in between each one, so the water will keep boiling. She scrapes up the chopped onions with the wide blade of a butcher knife and slides them into the melted butter in the frying pan. She can hear her mother scolding. "For Chrissake turn it down you're gonna burn the butter." Lucy always liked fieldwork better than housework with her mother pecking at her.

She's at the table finishing up the last bite of *kubasa*. Her place might be cramped, but it's better than those cardboard boxes the government builds for old people, that's for sure. When Phyllis pointed out that The Villa Suites were wheelchair-accessible, Lucy barked, "You think I wanna be with them church ladies? Listen to 'em cooing every time their grandkids stop by. You can probably hear your neighbour take a piss."

Her supper dishes are drying on a tea towel. In a TV ad for long-distance telephone, a little boy in a striped T-shirt and ball cap is sitting on his Grandma's lap. Lucy plucks a toffee from the Bargain Box of Assorted Chocolates and imagines if Phyllis had had a son, left him at the farm for the summer. Lucy would've shown him Chevs, Fords, and Oldsmobiles, so he'd know the difference. They would've built models on the kitchen table. They would've stood up the boxes with the picture of the finished projects, left out all the bits and the airplane glue till his next stay. When he was old enough, she would've taught him how to change the oil and do his own grease jobs. He would've called her Baba.

A grandson. That's what Lucy's imagining when she hears a siren. First a siren, then flashing lights. It's a police car. She burps up onions. When the headlights turn into Joy's driveway, Lucy wheels her chair around forty-five degrees. A second set of flashing lights. It's an ambulance. Acid rises in Lucy's throat. The chocolate-covered toffee is melting between her fingers. They'll see the bullet hole. Can't miss it.

Mary Had A Lamb

THREE FRESHLY BATHED WIDOWS IN PASTEL bathrobes and slippers, sit on their beds at the Holiday Inn Killarney. Mary in pink, Karen in mint green, Gail in yellow. Coloured Easter confections.

"When was the last time you had sex?" Mary asks.

"Where on earth did that question come from?" Karen looks up from her postcard, pen in hand. "I can't believe we're having this conversation. Let's see, it must have been '96, before Matt's prostate cancer and I'm glad to be finished with it. I can go to bed without getting felt up or poked."

Gail stops rubbing moisturizer into her feet. "The night before Richard died, if you must know. I've never told a soul. I still feel guilty to this day."

"Surely it couldn't have made any difference," is Mary's response. Now it's her turn. "Seven years ago for me. When Albert turned his eye toward men."

"What a bunch of losers we are," Karen comments. "Even nuns get a little nookie now and then. I'm turning in, girls."

Before falling asleep, Mary replays her wedding night with her first husband, George. She emerged from the steamy bathroom at the Centennial Motel and posed in a lacy peignoir set, mini-length. She was twenty years old and nervous. They embraced, climbed in between the sheets, turned off the light, undressed, French-kissed, and copulated. Going all the way took a total of five minutes. It would be several years until she experienced her first orgasm.

George died of a heart attack while Mary was in the garden, cutting a bouquet of peonies. They had been married twenty-one years. She continued to sleep on her half of the double bed, conjuring up the smell and feel of him.

After the children left home, a shiny British airman named Albert initiated Mary into the world of travel and martinis. He fussed over her bum, gave it a pet name. "Frilly, my plush pink pillow and mine alone," he would gush, caressing it with both hands. And Mary would counter with, "You devil!" Albert brought out the naughty in her. Thanks to his wide-ranging sexual repertoire, she came to understand the 69 logo screen-printed on T-shirts.

Mary was twitterpated by Albert. She streaked her hair and shopped for cocktail dresses. In bed, she whimpered and squealed, covering her mouth to silence screams. She hadn't screamed since she gave birth. They moved from Canada to England, where they played house for two years. She was charmed by the British ways and adored her new furniture courtesy of Albert's Royal Air Force pension, that is until he enlightened her on the concept of *bi*.

Mary returned to Canada by herself, and moved into a lavish retirement home. Grocery shopping, cooking, cleaning, and laundry became remnants of her past.

Now Mary takes pride in being (and looking) the youngest in her condo complex. Her Royal Doulton collection — *Soiree, Tess, My Love* — gleams behind glass in her china cabinet. From Monday to Thursday, she watches *All My Children* and reads Danielle Steele. Friday is the hairdresser, manicurist, electrolysis when needed, and a martini with an olive before dining alone. Saturday — lunch and a glass of wine with the girls. Sunday — church, a long afternoon nap, a dry martini in a crystal glass.

Gail and Karen, travel booklets in hand, pay Mary a visit one evening when she's tipsy. "We're thinking of going on a bus tour of Ireland," Gail begins. "Why don't you come along?"

Karen fills in details of the itinerary and the price for three sharing a room. "We'll draw straws to see who gets the rollaway cot."

That night in a dream, Mary falls under the spell of faeries from the tourist brochure.

The three women are in a queue at the Cork International Airport. "Look at those old broads with perms," Mary quips. "Permed hair, perma-press pantsuits, even perma-grins." Her own hair is chin length, salt and pepper, swingy.

Their tour host uses corny alliteration to help them learn one another's names. Gregarious Gail, Your Majesty Mary, K-K-K-Karen. Out of the corner of her mouth, Mary says, "She's grating on me and we've only been on this bus for half an hour."

Jumpin' Jack owns hotels in Boston and Tel Aviv, but now resides in London. For Lavender Lily from Vermont, it is the third trip to Ireland, the home of her ancestors, but the first since her husband's death. What they all have in common is a grudging acceptance of bus tours as their only travel option. They kibitz with one another, drink Guinness and eat soda bread, but do not delve into personal histories. Mary wonders when her tour-mates last had sex.

The host offers each of them a piece of bread as they exit the bus at Killarney National Park. "Put this in your pocket to ward off the faeries."

"You two enjoy the walk. My feet are throbbing." Mary shoos Gail and Karen along, then sits on a bench in the parking lot. The rush of the Torc Waterfall can be heard in the distance. After the group is out of sight, Mary feels drawn into the forest. One of several trails catches her attention. She follows it, her tender soles cushioned by the carpet of moss, as far as a conspicuous beech tree. Under its canopy, she stops to admire miniscule prisms created by sunlight on drops of mist.

"Thiss forest iss enchanted, y' know." The voice comes from a dark enclosure of ivy. In the hollow of a tree, Mary can discern a man wearing an emerald green frock coat with a ruffle around the neck and lace frills at his wrists. A park employee, perhaps a summer student, must have come up with this whimsical touch. Find a willing sod and pay him to dress up as a leprechaun to delight the tourists. She cannot help but smirk.

"I suppose you're a leprechaun." Judging from his diminutive little legs, Mary determines that he is no more than three feet tall, but she cannot be sure because he is seated on a stump.

"Yiss. The leprechaun of Killarney National Park." The tiny man has delicate features and a red beard. In Canada, his knee-length breeches, the goofy hat with a buckle, and the leather apron could be a Hallowe'en costume. "Making and mending shoes iss my vocation, but a lonely existence it iss." Beside his feet on the ground is a wrought-iron kettle. He's panhandling, Mary thinks. Throw a Euro in his pot o' gold and have your picture taken with a real live leprechaun.

"Come sit a minute, will ye?" The leprechaun points to another stump. "We sprites are approachable."

Mary is hesitant, but intrigued. She sits down six feet away from this strange creature. He uses a jackknife to shave off the worn edges of the sole of a work boot on his lap. Mary is taking it all in, his black stockings, his shiny pointed shoes the size of a child's.

"Liam O'Sullivan from Killarney I am. And yourself?"

The encounter is bizarre, but Mary cannot be rude to this little man. "Mary Fielding. I'm from Canada."

"Canada? Aye." Liam stitches the sole, all the while chattering about the little people of the forest, their goings-on and mishaps.

Mary finds his account to be novel, even alluring, sprinkled with words like "sylvans" and "nymphs".

"We are quite harmless ye know, though minor difficulties may occur."

When Mary stands to announce is time to meet her tour back at the bus, Liam looks directly into her eyes. She can feel her cheeks turn pink. After a silence, he asks boldly, "Would ye be givin' a man the pleasure of yeer company over a loavely dinner?"

When she does not reply, he adds, " . . . tomorrow eve at half seven?"

By the time Mary rejoins the group, she has disclosed the name of her hotel to the leprechaun and has accepted his dinner invitation. It all seems to have taken place quite naturally.

In the lobby of the Holiday Inn the next evening, Liam is wearing a pale blue shirt and dress pants with a pleat. He appears taller than Mary remembered, perhaps five feet eight inches. He is a lean man with boyish blue eyes, a dreamy look, and graying hair. He compliments Mary on her sweater as he reaches for her hand. "The colour red brings out the roses in yeer cheeks, Mary." He pronounces her name "May-ree", like a tenor at the end of a bar, holding a whole note, then clipping the quarter note. Not plain old "Merry".

Over cocktails and a candle, Liam asks, "*Ni he la na gaoithe la na scoilbe?* What good is a drink or a glass without the company that would put a taste on them?"

Mary does a self-conscious little shoulder shrug. This Irishman is almost as seductive as Albert. Beware, she cautions herself.

Liam has not taken his eyes off her. "Yeer skin iss like peaches and cream, Mary."

"It's probably the fresh air. I do a lot of walking back home."

"Irish women have ruddy complexions, have ye noticed?"

Their first glorious date ends with Liam pressing a moist and tender kiss on Mary's forehead as he wishes her *soft dreams* in the lobby of her hotel.

With a hurried explanation to the tour host, Mary plays hooky from the planned outings and instead follows Liam down faery paths lit by stardust. Her first overnight away from the hotel prompts a lecture from Karen and Gail, and the threat of informing her daughter.

"Ever since that day in the park, you've been distant," Gail chides. "Spacey. Like you're on drugs."

"We know it's a man," Karen adds. "But who is he and why haven't you introduced him to us? What if he's a lecher who preys on widows?"

Mary clicks her tongue. "His name is Liam O'Sullivan. My Lord, at the age of fifty-eight, do I have a curfew?" With the bus scheduled to depart for Cork in three days, Mary announces her decision to remain in Ireland.

Gail asks, "Have you lost your mind? It's as if you've fallen under a spell." To some extent, she is right. Mary feels as if she no longer belongs in their world. Speaking more loudly than necessary on the phone, with Gail hovering over her, Mary tells her daughter, "I was planning to call you, dear. I've met someone named Liam O'Sullivan and he's a real gentleman." Her voice is quavering. "A retired Sociology professor." She makes that up on the spot. "His wife died of cancer." That too. "We're very good together." She can't say she has discovered the girl she used to be or that this might be her last chance for romance and she isn't going to miss it.

A furnished self-catering apartment above a pub in the town of Kenmare is available for let. Mary pays three months rent in advance. On drizzly afternoons, under a feather tick, Liam melts into the softness of her body, overlooking the menopause pillow above her waist and the stretch marks below. His penis is more slender than George's and his testicles, covered in strawberry blonde curls, are smaller than Albert's. The size of meatballs. She nestles into Liam's shoulder until the coolness of the evening slips through the window. Liam is not like George, who held her after intercourse only until his breathing returned to normal and his bladder beckoned. As for Albert, he was too lustful for cuddling.

The Found Out Café is Liam and Mary's mid-morning coffee stop. Words of wisdom called *A Spoonful Of Irish* are printed on packets of sugar. To Mary, the first one is like the fortune in a fortune cookie. "*Is in aimsear an ghadhtar sea a nitear na cairde.* It's in the time of want that friends are made." In the afternoons, they tour County Kerry in a hire car, Liam entertaining Mary with a running commentary while she negotiates the narrow serpentine roads. In the evenings, Liam spins yarns about faeries, the deities of woods and waterfalls.

Mary queries him about his wrought-iron kettle, hoping the hint might prompt him to pay some of the food bills. His response is, "A rainbow emanates from my pot o'gold, Mary. It's my means of travel." She has yet to witness this phenomenon.

On a sunny afternoon, they return to the enclosure in Killarney National Park where they first met. Mary watches with disbelief as Liam takes on a luminous appearance. Her eyes widen when Poof! he decreases to his leprechaun height. "When ye first catch sight of us, we appear small," he explains, "but when ye've succumbed to our charm, we're as tall as humans." His rosebud mouth curls into an impish smile. "That would be Yeats."

The edges of the forest merge into one another, then recede into the distance. "Come with me to the Isle of Happiness, May-ree. Faerieland can be reached only through adventure, trials, spells, or love."

Liam leads her into an enchanted haven and gestures for her to undress. "I promise to make your little lamb bleat." Ever so slowly, the top of his head at her belly-button, his tongue perfectly situated, he whispers, "Your most sacred place." Liam keeps his promise, the juices of his lips bending her forward, her fingers gripping his scalp. Lying together in the moss afterward, his sweat takes on an earthy pungency. "I so wished to please ye here in this very place, Mary. Ye've become a woodland lover."

"Is that an official tourist designation? Will I get a badge, like when I kissed the Blarney Stone?"

"No badge, m'love, but ye'll be showin' me a little gratitude."

They lie naked and entwined, Mary feeling no self-consciousness, only a sense of freedom, wafts of warm air kissing her buttocks beneath the blue Irish sky.

When something, perhaps an insect, brushes against her eyelids, she sits up. "What was that? Are those butterflies?"

"You're close. Those are Pillywiggins, the smallest elves in the netherworld. If ye listen carefully, ye'll hear them hum while they're gatherin' honey."

"Pillywiggins?"

"Pillywiggins do exist, May-ree Fielding. They intermarry with the dragon flies and take good care of the smallest of flora and fauna. It's their job so. Aye, these woods they're inhabited by all sizes and shapes of the ancient creatures."

Mary begins dressing. "Have they been watching?"

"Yes. They delight in love-making."

Spring drifts into summer, then fall. Mary pays the rent, one month after another. When she marvels at the subtle change of seasons in Ireland, Liam claims that sprites make and unmake the seasons. He reads to her from Yeats in bed at night. "Faeries can only appear as borrowed forms that are within the limits of our awareness." Some of Yeats' stories are about ghosts traipsing around the earth at free will and others are about the solitude of age, but it is Yeats' love poetry that snags Mary's heart. "Why should I seek for love or study it? Were I but crazy for love's sake? Why does my heart beat so?"

Liam carries two leather pouches in the pockets of his pants. Mary, conscious of her bank balance dwindling and of Liam never once paying for anything, finds the right moment to ask him about the pouches. He readily opens one and takes out a silver shilling. If he spends this coin, it will return to the pouch by magic. The gold coin in the other pouch, he alleges, is for bribing his way out of difficult situations. He reminds Mary that leprechauns are afraid of being abducted by humans. Should that happen to him, he will give the gold coin to his kidnapper with the promise of great wealth if he is allowed to go free. After his escape, the gold coin will turn to ashes. Mary reaches for her purse and takes out some Euros. The coins seem both foreign and irrelevant to Liam, who dismisses her concerns over money. "Ye'll be plenty rich one day," he says. In the meantime, presumably she will continue to bear the financial responsibility for their tryst.

Mary awakens one misty moisty morning to find Liam lying quietly facing her. "Were you watching me sleep?" she asks. "I must be quite a sight. Puffy eyes and drool."

"A pretty sight ye are in my eyes, May-ree Fielding. I was embroidering your thoughts so." My, he could be capricious.

"You're a poet, Liam, and I love you for it."

A chilly northwest wind gusts down the Henry Street corridor, practically pulling the door out of Liam's hand as they step into the Found Out Café. At Mary's request, the server gives her a packet of sugar with her Americano. It reads, "*Is glas iad cnoic i bfad uainn*. Far away hills are green." When she broaches the subject of the future, Liam's response is, "Time does not exist, Mary." He quotes Yeats for back-up. "Time drops in decay."

That might be true for Liam O'Sullivan and for William Butler Yeats, but the passage of time is real for Mary. She has missed her grandson's high school graduation in Canada. Her daughter has been pestering her for a photo of her boyfriend, but how can Mary oblige when Liam appears as a leprechaun in pictures? Her tears flow easily and often. She is struggling to preserve the link between this world and the other.

Collared doves coo, stirring Mary from her dreams. An early morning mist shrouds the town of Kenmare. She puts on the kettle for tea as usual, but this particular morning has a different feel. "Liam?" He isn't in the bathroom. "Liam?" Or the living-groom. Where has he gone so early? She calls his name again, as if expecting him to appear by magic.

After an interminable day of waiting with her stomach doing flip-flops, she decides to call her daughter. It will be afternoon in Canada. Beside the telephone on the bedside table, Mary discovers Liam's gold coin. What does this mean? She squeezes it in the palm of her hand while she talks. "No real reason, I just felt lonesome for you, dear." Surely her daughter can detect the strain in her voice. "Christmas? I haven't decided."

Mary paces, lies down, stands up, heats leftover soup but can't swallow it, deliberates over the future, repeatedly sits on the toilet, flips through a newspaper, takes a bath, puts on her kimono, watches the few passersby under the street lights. Her gut tells her Liam has returned to his forest glade and he will not be coming back. Mary phones her daughter a second time. "All right, book my flight. I'm coming home for Christmas." When she places the telephone on its cradle on the bedside table, the gold coin is gone and in its place is a tiny puddle of ashes. Did Liam feel entrapped by her? Or has he left so she could go home? He did say faeries can decide one's fate.

Holiday romances are not meant to last. Mary will dearly miss Liam's musty scent, his voice reading poetry, and his peculiar ideas, but the memory of him will remain as sparkling as gossamer. She leans forward and, with one breath, the ashes vanish into the air.

The Irish Tenors croon through speakers in the Quills Store while Mary chooses Christmas presents for her family — a linen tablecloth, a Donegal tam, mohair rugs, a felt purse. On display among souvenirs is a black plastic pot o'gold in clear cellophane wrap dotted with green shamrocks. The pot o'gold is filled to the brim with gold foil-covered chocolate coins.

"Were I but crazy for love's sake?" Yes.

"Why should I seek for love or study it?" Why not?

Windy Height

AMELIA O'DEA HAS LIVED SEVEN LIFETIMES on the wild and craggy tip of the Beara Peninsula, so long that her spirit has fused with the landscape. She is the old woman of Beara, *An Cailleach Beara*.

To Amelia, the need for a cable car to Dursey Island is a mystery. It is Ireland's only cable car and attracts tourists following the Ring of Beara. While they wait for their ten-minute ride, they snap photos of the sign: "ATTENTION. You may be required to relinquish your seat should a sheep from Dursey Island be in need of a veterinarian." They board the cable car and dangle over Bantry Bay until they reach the more-or-less-uninhabited Dursey Island (Population: 6). Those who have the good fortune to share passage with a sheep and a shepherd never mind the stench. It is a tourist's dream, photos to show friends back home how quaint and old-fashioned Ireland is at the end of the twentieth century.

To Seán Quinn, the cable car to Dursey Island is a paycheque and a means to remain on the Beara Peninsula, unlike his classmates who have emigrated to Australia or Canada to find work. Seán drives twenty minutes from Castletownbere each morning to perform his duties as the operator of the cable car. And each evening, he returns home to his perky bride, Josie, who smothers him with kisses, runs his bath, and tickles him under the bottom edge of the towel he wraps around his burly self.

It is Josie's idea to open a bed and breakfast on undeveloped land adjacent to the cable station. She has searched the title of the property to ensure there are no liens, and has approached the owner, who is willing to sell. B & B's are trendy in Ireland's burgeoning tourist industry, especially in Josie's home province of Leinster, and bank financing is readily available (too much so) during The Celtic Tiger.

Josie envisions visitors from England and the United States, perhaps even Canada or Japan, returning on the last run from Dursey Island at 5:30 PM, and being served an evening meal. Her fantasy encompasses a sunroom, a vegetable garden, an assortment of animals in pens, and the promise of a wee *baibin*.

Seán's father gives the parcel of land to them for a wedding present after Seán tells him of *their* plans. "He's a generous man, me Da, buying us that land," Seán says to Josie, and she snaps back, not wasting a second to rein in her tongue, "Sure why would he not, and yourself the only son."

Homemaking in a one-bedroom flat in Castletownbere while Seán is away at the cable car is simply boring for Josie. Some days, she rides along with him and spends the day exploring their land. Josie loves their parcel of land. For her, it was love at first sight. She loves the wildness, but intends to tame it. She loves the idea of shaping it, making it her own, like she will tame and shape her new husband — polish his dull spots, teach him manners, correct his grammar. Coach him to shave, to scrub his face and clean his ears and change into a clean shirt when visitors are expected. To stay home with her on Friday nights instead of growing old with pint in hand at O'Dwyer's Tavern like one of the town's bachelors. Sure, he's great *craic* when he has a few pints on him, but it's time he acted like a married man.

On one of her tagalong-with-Seán days, Josie is determined to find a route that leads to the seashore on their land. After she and Seán share the lunch she packed, she has four hours left for exploring. She follows a rutted sheep path zigzagging its way through bracken, but before she reaches the sea, the path intersects with a much narrower track. Curious about where that track might lead, Josie turns and proceeds in an easterly direction. To put one foot in front of the other through cow parsley and furze requires concentration, so she is startled when she looks up and sees, directly in her path, a hovel she did not know existed. It is not visible from the road or from the prospective site for her B & B.

A weathered old woman pokes her head out of the door of the hovel. Josie has no choice but to introduce herself now that she has been seen. She feels a stitch of disquiet because she does not know exactly where their property ends and the neighbours' begins. Perhaps she is trespassing. The woman, with a black shawl over her yellowing hair, steps out and closes the door behind her, but not before Josie has glimpsed a dark interior and inhaled smouldering turf.

"Rain again today," Josie begins, her bobbling earrings synchronized with the nodding of her head.

The shawlie fusses to straighten her saggy grey jumper with a longer navy jumper over top, and her charcoal wool skirt with an uneven hemline. Two large safety pins are fastened over her flat bosom. Her eyes dart between the trespasser's shoes and her own, then settle on the dirt packed hard against the door sill.

Josie pokes at her own sternum and says, "Josephine Quinn".

When the woman does not respond, Josie increases her volume and enunciates, "I'm . . . Josie . . . Quinn . . . And . . . what . . . would . . . your . . . name . . . be?"

The woman straightens her back, looks up, and states, "Amelia O'Dea". She has no teeth, and kinky white hairs sprout in all directions from her chin.

"I'm . . . sorry . . . for . . . any . . . bother . . . or . . . if . . . I . . . startled . . . you, Amelia O'Dea." Josie surveys the scrap of scrub land without moving her feet, noting Amelia's well and privy, her turfpile, and a trough possibly used for pigs in the past. Josie asks Amelia her age and how long she has lived there, but Amelia says she can't remember.

Josie chatters about the wind and the spring season, then apologizes again. "I'm sorry for the bother," turns and adds, "I'll be leaving you alone so."

On her way back up the jagged cliff, it occurs to Josie that what she has just seen is beyond belief — Amelia herself and the shack, not much better than a famine house, leaning away from the sea. Josie drives to Waterford, back to the Land Registry, where an officious clerk pecks with manicured nails on a computer keyboard. Josie asks if the property has ever been owned by anyone by the name of O'Dea and is told that no such record exists.

"What if, hypothetically speaking, there was a squatter on a piece of land, what might the owner do?"

The clerk informs her of the legal protocol for evicting squatters. Being of good Catholic conscience, Josie has no intention of evicting the frail Amelia or collecting rent, but her charity will not extend to upgrading Amelia's cottage or clearing the overgrown path. Besides, the cottage may not even be on their land. The property markers are most likely concealed by plant growth.

Josie's instincts tell her that the old woman, so shy and wild, must remain unknown. On the drive home, she makes a decision not to tell Seán about Amelia, for fear of him changing his mind about proceeding with the land transaction. It will be the first, but not the only secret, she keeps from him.

Eoin O'Farrell, the shepherd of Dursey Island, once climbed that path each week on his way to Allihies to purchase provisions. His eyes were drawn to Amelia's breasts taking womanly shape. She would be hoeing the hard soil between rows of potatoes and turnips that would, *dia toilteanach*, merciful God, see her and her parents through winter. Without stopping, Eoin would say to Amelia's father seated on a bench, "Rain again today."

On summer evenings, Eoin abandoned his shepherdly duties, traversed the narrow sound, tied his *currach* to a rock, and hastened across the pebbly beach to meet Amelia. They would scramble up the steep cliff, breathing in the wild sweet alison, him following so close that her skirt whipped his pantlegs. Always there was wind. Often there was rain. They would walk hand-in-hand as far as the graveyard and make love in the rough meadow-grass between the last row of tombstones and the falling-down fence, their only privacy.

In July of 1936, giant waves caused by strong westerlies capsized Eoin O'Farrell's *currach* on his way back to Dursey Island after a rendezvous with Amelia. The flotsam that had been his boat washed up on the rocky shore, and Amelia, sixteen years old, saved the wreckage. It was all that remained of darling

Eoin, and for her there would be no other prodding tongue or furry groin in the long years ahead.

Amelia attended to the needs of her aging parents until their remains were carried by the neighbour men up the path and along the road to the graveyard, the place where she had loved Eoin. Cow parsley and furze flourished with the cycling of the seasons, and narrowed the rugged path to the width of two human feet.

The Quinns fence in a pen for sheep and a lama, and begin construction of their home, including a conservatory and separate entrance for B & B guests. While raking up carpenters' debris, Josie sees Amelia open the gate to their sheep pen, pet the animals, tut in Irish, close the gate, and trudge back home with long sheep's hairs and fresh manure on her skirt. She is not sure-footed, stumbling over furrows.

Josie is overwhelmed by her enterprise and gives little thought to Amelia or her needs. Never once has she passed the old woman walking on the gravel road carrying a sack of messages. By fall, their home is ready for occupancy. Finishing touches to the exterior will have to wait until next spring.

Seán appreciates the proximity to the cable car. He can even come home for lunch and MCT. That's what Josie has coined their amorous daylight performances — "Mutual Cuddling Time." Wind gusts are common, at times approaching hurricane force, and Seán is shouldered with the responsibility of deciding when it is hazardous to operate the cable car.

Josie capitalizes on this meteorological phenomenon, naming her bed and breakfast "Windy Height". She writes up an advert for tourism publications and websites: "Stay at *Cnoc Gaofar* Windy

Height B & B, with a view of Bantry Bay and Dursey Island. Stunning cliffs for birdwatching. Situated close to the cable car."

She invites two other couples for Christmas dinner, in part to show off her home, as young wives are known to do. As she is telling her guests about her plans for the opening of her bed and breakfast in May, Amelia makes an appearance. She hovers next to the sideboard where Josie has arranged six small plates, each with a slice of blackberry pie and a dessert fork. Amelia's ankles are swollen and her shoes have taken on the form of her misshapen feet. Neither Seán nor their guests acknowledge Amelia. They do not stare at her layered wool garments, her shawl, or the safety pins holding her jumper together where buttons have gone missing.

When Josie clears the dinner plates and stacks them on the sideboard, she brushes against Amelia. Hopefully, her body odour will be masked by the pine-scented candles and the cinnamon sticks simmering in cider.

Josie's cheeks are flushed, not from the wine alone, and her speech is over-excited as she serves the pie. Amelia reaches for morsels of lamb left on the plates, and crumbs of pastry on the crocheted doily. But when she uses her fingernails to dig out the mush compacted between her dentures, and the hairs on her chin bristle, Josie is repulsed and has to look away.

A winter draft kisses Josie's ankles under the table. She thinks Amelia must have let herself out, so she hurries into the kitchen on the pretext of making more tea and there, on the doorstep, stands Amelia. Josie begs her to wait right there. She returns with a small package of leftover leg of lamb, blackberry pie, and a flashlight. Amelia points to the moon and says, "*Lochran aigh nam boch*". The lamp of the poor. And she is on her way.

Josie takes a few deep breaths to calm herself and resumes her role as hostess, refilling china teacups. She waits for a lull in the Christmas reminiscing to interject, "The girl at the Land Titles Office was mentioning people by the name of O'Dea used to live along this road."

Seán is quick to correct her. "Nah, Josephine, there's been no O'Deas on Beara that I've ever heard of."

One of the other husbands adds, "Maybe 'twas *An Cailleach* the girl was speaking of," and laughs.

Then the five of them, all a drop taken, share the in-joke, reminding Josie that she's *from away*. Josie springs to her feet and collects the stack of dinner plates. Seán, noticing the shiny tips of her earlobes and her mottled throat, catches her around the waist and pulls her close. He loves her short fuse, her inability to camouflage her emotions. He buries his face in her midriff, in her slippery red Christmas blouse, all the while concocting a persuasive scenario for seducing her after their guests leave, to hell with tidying up. He can go beyond her perfume to inhale the smell of her. She knows what he's up to and would smack him if her arms weren't full. Instead she wriggles free and goes through the door into the kitchen.

Neither of the wives lifts a finger. At the table, they carry on with the men poking fun at old superstitions and reciting poems they were forced to memorize in primary school.

"*Ebb-tide has come to me as to the sea. Old age makes me yellow.*"

"*It is riches you love, and not people. As for us, when we lived, it was people we loved.*"

Josie catches the tail end of it, one of the wives saying, " . . . walking home from catechism and someone would whisper '*An Cailleach Beara*' and we'd all be running up the boreen and through the first unlocked door, squealing with fright. Look now, I've goosebumps just talking about it."

And, before changing the subject, Seán adds, "Tis no more than old people's talk. *Seafóid*. Nonsense. Belongs in the dustbin is all."

Winter extends into late March. Snow showers continue to fall, isolating residents along Bantry Bay, those on the Beara Peninsula to the north and those on the Sheep's Head Peninsula to the south. Then, to demoralize them further, a hurricane (downgraded to an extratropical cyclone) batters Co. Cork. Heavy rainfall and winds increasing in fury to gale force damage buildings, down trees, and result in flooding and chaos on the roadways. Josie huddles indoors, leaving it to Seán to oversee their place, their animals, and their vehicle. When she sees on RTE News that eleven deaths have been reported in Ireland and the UK, she decides she had better check on Amelia after the storm blows itself out. She has spotted the shawlie only one time since Christmas, poking a handful of grass through the wooden slat fence into the mouth of their lama. That must have been in February.

It is mid-April when Josie screws up her courage. The prospect of discovering a decomposed body gives her the creeps. She worries if Amelia were to die on their property, might they bear some responsibility?

She sets out, but comes to a stop when the path disappears. It has folded in on itself, leaving a ridge like the puckered scar from an abdominal incision, with flesh pleated on either side. Josie tramples cow parsley and blue-green spikes of furze, clearing a passageway down the hill to the cottage, with its roof caved in, and meadow-grass beginning to sprout. The peninsula has wrapped the old woman of Beara in a blanket of earth and has laid her to rest.

Tres Leches

Thrilled

ONE WOMAN'S LIFETIME OF JEWELLERY IN a pink satin nest — a souvenir bracelet from New York City, a heart with a red rose alongside "Mother", a rhinestone brooch in the shape of a pinwheel — treasures befitting a Woolworth's jewellery box, its lid resting at an angle. Morsels are jammed in the bottom compartment — extra buttons, Samsonite keys, broken clasps, widowed earrings. The daughter inherits her mother's jewellery. Chicken feed. The son inherits the farm.

From the chiffonier, baggy stockings, brassieres held together with safety pins, nylon slips, underpants with dangling elastic, and yellowed nighties go straight into a wastebasket. Grace singles out never-used towels from across the line and flowered pillowcases still in J.C. Penney packages. Too good to give away. She discards the housedresses from the dusty, stale, narrow closet. The good dresses, now out of style, are destined for the church rummage sale.

Pauline was a morning person. She got up at sunrise, whatever time the sun rose. It wasn't because she was eager to read or do a crossword puzzle or even get started on her housework. She simply greeted the dawn. In summer, she stood on the grass in her duster and slippers and looked up at the sky. In winter, she pulled on a pair of ski-doo boots and any old jacket hanging in the porch. One of Johann's caps covered her head on rainy mornings. Sometimes she went back to bed and got up again at a sensible hour. Johann never questioned her. What was important to him after morning chores was porridge and coffee, both with sugar and cream.

Grace leaves the top drawer for last. *Kjinja* had been told to keep their noses out, but when Pauline was weeding the garden or butchering chickens, young Gracie snooped. Her mother always kept a ten and a twenty-dollar bill tucked in her German Bible. Pin money? Emergency money? Her own money? Inside the back cover, she had written the birthdates of her children. Lillian, Anna, Edgar, Grace. Grace would always be the baby.

Bundled together with white sewing elastic tied in a bow are old letters, birthday cards, and obituaries. Fancy embroidered handkerchiefs and a *Sisters Forever* charm are saved in their original flat cardboard boxes. Presents from Aunt Beatrice, "Bee-ah".

The black leather cover of *Das Volga Gesang-Buch* is embossed with "Pauline Engel" in gold script. Between onionskin pages after Hymn 345, "*O Jesu Christe, wahres Licht*" is a lacy handkerchief. Folded inside is a string of tiny glass beads.

On days when Grace stayed home from school fake-sick, she was allowed in her parents' bed on the main floor. She would take her mother's jewellery box into bed and, with pillows propped behind her back, would try on the necklaces and clip-on earrings and admire her little white face in the hand mirror from the tortoise shell dresser set. Once, when Pauline came to feel Gracie's forehead, she caught her standing by the open drawer with the string of glass beads in her hand. It was the only time Grace ever saw her mother blush.

"Sophia."

"*Donner Waada noch emol*, Pauline. Who is this Sophia you're always talking about? We don't know any Sophia. What kind of name is that anyway?" Johann touched her tight lips with a red plastic spoon. "Here, have some ice cream before it melts. We'll change the subject. That's a good girl. Remember when I used to stop at the Dairy Queen on the way home from church? I'd buy us strawberry sundaes."

"*Ach*, that was nothing." She looked straight at him with her rheumy eyes. "I was the one who had to get up early to make sure dinner was ready."

"*Nah yah*, but you had a good life, *Pauline-je*. Remember the time we went down East to pick up a new car? One more bite. *En bätje.*"

Coarse dark hairs trembled on Pauline's upper lip.

"*Scheenschmakt?* And the Black Hills, the Passion Play? You were in your glory shopping in Minot."

"And don't forget Gracie took me to New York."

"*Yah. Ach du lieber Augustine!*"

"You rang the bell, Mr. Schmidt?"

"Pauline made a puddle."

"We'll have that fixed up in no time, won't we darling?"

Pauline hiked up her skirt, exposing the droopy skin on her thighs, and a diaper.

Johann abruptly stood up. "I'll leave you two girls alone. I was just about to go anyhow." He bent down to kiss Pauline on the forehead. A duty-kiss.

With her eyes squeezed shut, tears leaked down either side of her red nose.

Covered with a thin green blanket, talcum powder on her bottom, Pauline whispered "Sophia" to nobody. On the screen of her closed eyelids, Sophia appeared, sitting cross-legged on the ground nursing a baby, her burgundy nipple full and wet. Johann would be having his *Meddach schlop* in the La-Z-Boy, a worn thing. After his nap, he'd heat up a half-can of Campbell's tomato soup and make himself a fried egg sandwich for supper, listen to the CBC Radio news. His bachelor routine.

Every door along the institutional hallway was identical except for a laminated sign with the occupant's name and photo outlined by a cheery computer-generated border. The photo of Pauline, head slumped forward, milky eyes behind bifocals, was bordered by mauve tropical lavinia. *Aloha!* After Pauline died, the matron gave the poster to Grace, together with a green garbage bag filled with Pauline's personal effects. As if she wanted a souvenir of the nursing home where her mother had spent the last seven years of her life.

Face black beneath the cap line, Johann stomped his boots on the mat and opened his red polka-dot hanky to show Pauline the saskatoons. She placed a berry on her tongue and smacked her mouth open and closed, assessing its flavour and juiciness. "Just right for jam. I'm going berry picking tomorrow."

"It's a long walk in your condition."

"*Ach*, I have strong *dietsche* legs, remember?"

Ankle socks, bare legs with a fine web of hairs, a brown scarf tied at the nape, and long sleeves for protection from scratchy branches. In a pail she carried a quart sealer of water, meat between slices of brown bread, and two gingersnaps. Johann grasped the fencepost with his forearm, sliding the loop of barbed wire up and over the post to open the gate for Pauline. Heidi, a collie of sorts, slopped drool on his pantleg.

The flora in the cow pasture did not attract Pauline's attention. In the Big House where she grew up, there had been no talk of fragrant yarrow or delicate needle-and-thread grass, but she had learned how long to crank the churn before spooning butter into a press. She may not have known that the meadow dressed differently for each season, but when she cut lard into the dry ingredients for pie pastry, she could *riffle* the crumbs just so. Hoary puccoon and goat's beard were irrelevant, but if you asked her how many times to sift Robin Hood flour to make a fine-textured white cake, she could have told you. The knee-high grass, wet with morning dew, cooled her legs.

Crossing the ploughed field, her shoes filled with powdery dirt. Oat plants standing like little soldiers in straight rows were six inches high. "A nice rain would make them happy," she said out loud.

As she neared the bush, house sparrows took flight, telescoping to black specks like pepper sprinkled upwards into the sky. A pair of striped chipmunks scurried away, one chasing the other. Clusters of berries weighed down the high branches of the saskatoon bushes. She set her pail on the ground, pulled a branch toward her, and with just the right firmness to her grip, stripped the ripe berries, leaving behind the red ones and the green ones. She did not hear the lark buntings' whistles, interspersed with rattles and trills, nor the *cheerily, cheer up, cheer up, cheerily, cheer up* of the robins. Only the buzzing of flies. *I hope Bea isn't making a mistake marrying Bernie,* she was thinking. *His job is only till harvest and then what? They could wind up in the poorhouse.* Handfuls of saskatoons pinged on the steel pail until the bottom was covered. She worked her way through the bush, berry-picking and swatting at mosquitoes with a switch torn from a willow bush. *Supper? Smoked sausage and new potatoes. There was still some homemade cheese, Je koakte kjees, in the icebox and a couple of pieces of Aupel'kuake. Anna,* she thought she'd like to call the baby Anna if it was a girl, but Johann wanted to name it after his sister Lillian.

From the shadows came a disturbance, scuffling, twigs snapping. *Could it be a deer? Pauline would love to see one close-up. Could it be a coyote?* Her neck and shoulders tightened at the prospect. A torrent of goose bumps rushed from her head to her toes. She had not spied any of those devils skulking around her chicken coop since Johann had brought the pup home from the neighbour's.

One instant she heard rustling in the underbrush, her head turned toward the sound, her eyes located its source, and the next instant . . . recognition. That's how it happened. *Gott in Himmel, en Mäakje!*

Accompanied by faint tinkling, a dark girl popped up from a shady patch, her mustard-coloured blouse slipping from one shoulder. Her amiable smile and the jaunty little bob of her head conveyed the notion that she had every right to be there. Her soot-black hair was tied back, with wilful curls escaping from behind her ears. Her earrings must have been two inches long with fine chains on the ends quivering like tassels. Pauline stood her ground. The girl broke the impasse with, "*So cero nay?*" She placed the palm of one small hand flat to her chest and said "Sophia" with a sprightly giggle, then pointed to Pauline. Her nostrils flared perceptibly. My she was bold for such a scrawny thing.

Pauline was timid by nature, but in this encounter deliberately guarded. How could she welcome a trespasser on Johann's land? "I'm Pauline" was her response in a cool tone of voice. What kind of name is Sophia? she wondered. She was not from sturdy stock, that's for sure. Just a little bit of a thing, probably caught every sickness that went around. And so oddly dressed. On such a warm day, to be wearing a finger-pleated skirt down to the ground?

Sophia's inquisitive black eyes darted from Pauline's face to her pregnant belly and she spoke in a language Pauline could not decipher. With childish impulsivity, Sophia approached until they were only arms' length apart, then reached out the fingertips of one hand to Pauline's *Schwellung*. My she was froward. Pauline averted her gaze.

"Baby," said the girl in a voice high and sweet. She took Pauline's stiff and reluctant hand and placed it on her own stomach. Pauline was not in the habit of touching strangers below the waist, never mind a half-breed. Her fingers, as if of their own volition, nevertheless relaxed and moulded to a roundness under the red, purple, and black threads woven into the fabric of Sophia's skirt. She was not a *En Mäakje* after all, she was a *Fru*. Her lips, lush and brown, were in motion, chattering away like a chipmunk. Where on earth had this curious *Auslanderin* come from? Pauline's armpits were damp, her cheeks flushed, and her breathing shallow. Following Sophia's lead, she took her lunch out of her pail. In the shade of a poplar bluff, the two women stretched out their legs, leaning against tree trunks, and ate.

"*Woa fon Kjemst du?*" Pauline posed the question, but couldn't make out Sophia's response. Sophia's habit of laughing at the end of every sentence amused Pauline. She chirped, but her laugh was husky. A beguiling combination.

It seemed as if Sophia couldn't be still. The whole time she ate and talked, she wriggled on the ground, twisting and turning, crossing her legs, uncrossing them, then tucking them under her. She would gesture with her hands, tug on the neckline of her blouse, and end some sentences with a question mark, shrugging her shoulders. She would brush her hair back with her fingers and lift her ponytail off her neck, then plop it back down again. Complementing all of this fidgeting was a sporadic delicate tinkle. Pauline sat stolid as a *Klumpen* of laundry soap. No longer wary, she could not help but delight in the performance.

Sophia reached into her paper lunch bag and offered Pauline a strip of something that looked like tanned cowhide. Pauline politely placed the end of it on her tongue, expecting a meaty flavour, but to her surprise, the taste was of molasses. She twisted off a bite-sized piece and began chewing to soften it. It occurred to her to offer Sophia a gingersnap in return. The tangy cookie prompted Sophia's eyes to widen and her head to nod as if to say, "*Sea goot! Danke.*" Both drank from sealers of water, warm by midday.

Sophia's saskatoons were piled on a square of striped cloth beside her. Her prattle continued as she rose onto her knees, brought two corners of the cloth together, tied them in a knot, did the same with the other two corners, then bounced to her feet. She was getting ready to leave. She poked a long peeled stick though the knots and tied the ends one final time. The word *knapsack* came into Pauline's mind as Sophia rested the bundle on her bony shoulder.

"*Baxt hai sastimos tiri patragi,*" Sophia said. Perhaps they were words of farewell and good luck as if the encounter had meant something to her, too. She patted her stomach with one hand, fluttered her fingers in a wave, and ventured off, tinkling.

Pauline's eyes were riveted to this exotic *Fru's* narrow back, her frizzy ponytail swinging from side to side on the yellow of her blouse. In a matter of seconds, Sophia turned around and hurried back as if she'd forgotten something. When she lifted the hem of her skirt off the ground, the toes of her black leather slippers peeked out. She removed one string of tinkling glass beads from her slender ankle, and with this gift, transferred electrical sparks to the palm of Pauline's hand. The women's eyes met and softened, but neither spoke. Sophia floated away. Pauline watched, entranced, until she was out of view.

On the prairie, on an ordinary July day, Pauline Schmidt had glimpsed beauty. It was there for a moment and then it was gone, slipped through her fingers. Sophia was a delicate colourful butterfly out of a picture book. And Pauline, with her big bones, straight hair, and peasant garb was a moth. In her hand were the beads and in her bosom a soaring. Sophia was gone, but would return when Pauline soothed a colicky infant or sprinkled Paris Green on her cabbages, when she canned peaches or waxed the oilcloth floor. Sophia would appear while Pauline was feeding a pair of overalls through the wringer and coaxing them out of the other side into the rinse water. When Pauline lay in a nursing home covered with a thin green blanket, Sophia would be her companion.

Several times on the walk home, when Pauline stopped to transfer the pail from one hand to the other, she held her string of brightly coloured beads up to the sun. When she rolled one between her thumb and fingertip, her angle of view changed and the bead spangled. It was transformed from deep saffron to yellow to orange. She tucked the beads back into her sock. Oh, she could hardly wait to tell Johann about Sophia. For once, she had something more than gossip from *koffe' klautsch* at the Big House.

Sausage *spretsed* in the frying pan. New potatoes steamed until they burst their skins. Picking over the saskatoons for jam, Pauline imagined Sophia untying her knapsack to show her husband the berries. He would close his eyes and open his mouth. She would place one on his tongue, then close her own eyes and open her mouth. He would place two or three on her tongue. The exchange would increase in volume and speed until they would be stuffing fists full of saskatoons into each other's mouths, chewing and swallowing and laughing with mouths wide open, lips and teeth purple, unashamed of their appetite.

At the table, Pauline mustered her courage to tell Johann about Sophia. "Today in the bush . . . " Every time, he interrupted or she lost her nerve. How would he react? Would he think she was foolish being friendly to an intruder? She listened with half an ear to his talk of roofing.

In bed, their conversation was of The Fair the next day. His calloused hand reached over to rest on her thigh. *"Goot owend."* Chirps of crickets drifted in, then faint strains of fiddles. Could it possibly be fiddles?

Johann spit out the word "Gypsies", followed by *"Dratjijch"*. Dirty Gypsies. "They're camping by the slough. *Ach*, they'll be peddling their pots and pans at the fair. And their black magic. I'll have to keep an eye on my horses." She heard his derisive snort.

Pauline lay with her eyes wide, the heavens dotted with stars outside the small, high bedroom window. She listened to a spirited melodeon in the distance. A broody man, his hair greased back, was kissing Sophia, she knew it. Kissing her without restraint under the aurora borealis. *Des Polarlichts*. That very moment, lying in bed, she knew she would never tell Johann about Sophia. She would need a hiding place for the beads. A reverie of sweet music and romance put her to sleep.

She stirred at sunrise as always, then relapsed into a dream of ruby red and purple. The *Maltj* cow was bawling, impatient to be milked. When she was fully awake, she stepped outside to greet the day, then hurried back in to reach for the beads under her pillow. Sophia was real. The old *Grünthal* General Store came into Pauline's memory, the time *Mutter* took her by the shoulders and gave her a good shake, then threatened to sell her to the gypsies if she didn't behave. The scolding did not evoke fear as intended, but rather mystery. Gypsies? Who are the gypsies?

"Pauline." A chubby nurse's aide with garlic breath was awakening her.

Sophia is dancing in a meadow, her hair untamed. Her husband, in a red silk shirt with billowing sleeves, draws his bow across the strings of a fiddle. His left hand quivers on the fingerboard and he leans in a rolling motion, feet digging into the grass. So tender is the music. He pauses, then dips. Scroll pointed down, he strikes the strings with the stick of the bow *col legno*, one, two, three times, then tips it back up, sweet again.

"Pauline," the nurse's aide repeated. "We need to go potty before supper. Try to roll over onto your side, okay?" As Pauline was being helped onto the toilet, she let out a loud crisp fart and both women laughed. "When I was a new bride, I had to put up with Johann's *futses* in a one-room shack."

"Honestly, men can be such pigs."

"What's for supper?"

"A fruit plate. Cottage cheese, peaches and toast. Canned peaches, of course."

"Canning peaches," Pauline mumbled. The wood stove in the cellar. She was about to preserve a case of Freestone peaches from the Okanagan. The water had come to a boil in navy blue kettles speckled with white. Sweat dripped off her forehead as she began blanching the peaches.

"Hotter than Hell," Pauline said as the nurse's aide wheeled her down the corridor. In her mind, she had been scalding quart sealers and metal lids with red chapped hands. She had turned to Gracie, who was dressing her dolly, and said, "Don't ever get married, *meine Kjinja*. Run off with the gypsies."

The pinwheel brooch brings back Christmas Eve — Jap oranges, *O Tannenbaum*, the floor littered with toys and mitts, white figure skates, ripped cardboard boxes and wrapping paper. It's almost time for *Wienachtowendate* — fried farmer's sausage, white buns, and sugary *riffle Kuchen* — every bite homemade. Before her mother drifts off to the kitchen to don a *Husfru* apron, her father appears with a small package wrapped in red foil, a gift Gracie happens to know was not under the tree. Proud as the Magi bearing pretend-gold, frankincense, and myrrh in the Sunday School pageant, he holds his offering out in front in both hands and walks toward Pauline. He bends down to kiss her smack-dab on the lips and bestow his offering. *"Froehliche Weihnachten,* my dear."* Quick as a wink, Gracie is beside her mother.

Pauline painstakingly detaches the pouffy gold bow first, then runs her stubby thumbnail along the Scotch tape, removes the paper and irons it out with her hand. Gracie can tell she's planning to save the wrapping paper and bow for next Christmas. "Park's Jewellery" reveals itself on a royal blue box. Pauline lifts a velvet case out of the box and unhinges its lid. Inside is a sparkly rhinestone brooch and earrings in the shape of pinwheels. The velvet box has been designed especially to fit the three pieces. Grace is leaning against her mother's soft shoulder.

"Try it on, *Pauline-je.* They call it aurora borealis. *Des Polarlichts"*

She puts on the earrings. *"Ach,* these are too fancy for me."

"Nä. I want my wife to look good."

Her upper lip dents in, a trait of her smile, but her heart isn't in it. Oh, she'll wear the jewellery to twenty-fifth anniversaries and Johann's Lions Club banquets, but she isn't an aurora-borealis-kinda-girl.

Grace imagines her father at Park's Jewellery. Mr. Park would have been at his desk poring over an open accounting ledger while overseeing his salesgirl chit-chatting with Johann. "Aurora borealis is all the rage this year," she would say. "The great thing about rhinestones is that they're iridescent. They take on whatever colour a lady is wearing." To prove her point, she would have held the brooch next to her blue blouse, then rested it on a red velvet pillow. "See?"

With the demeanour of prosperity, her father would have declared, "You've made a sale," without even asking the price. Mr. Park would have risen from his desk to accept the large bill her father pulled out of his wallet. The two men would have talked about snowfall, taxes, and John Diefenbaker. It was about time the West had a voice in Ottawa. The salesgirl would have cut the heavy foil paper deftly, wrapped the box with polished nails, Scotch-taped it, and attached a gold bow. The whole performance in a flash. Mr. Park would have shaken Grace's father's hand. "Merry Christmas, Johann. And a prosperous New Year." Beaming with glossy lipstick, the salesgirl would have said in a breathy voice, "Your wife will be thrilled. Merry Christmas."

Before Grace tucks the string of beads back into the lacy handkerchief, she holds it up to the square of sunlight in her parents' bedroom window. She rolls one of the tiny glass beads between her thumb and fingertip. As her angle of view changes, the bead spangles. It is transformed from deep saffron to yellow to orange.

Lunch at the Empire State Building

GRACIE SAID WHY WASTE MONEY. A hostel isn't my idea of a holiday, but I gave in, didn't want to start off on the wrong foot. She insists we're going Dutch. Guess she wants to prove she's all grown up.

Me on a bottom bunk with Gracie on the top and two other sets of bunks with four strangers in the same room, I can hardly believe it myself. In the bathroom down the hall, wet hairs weave in and out of the floor drain in the shower. Good thing I packed my rubber shoes. The cleaning lady must have to pull out those mats of hair, not to mention the long black hairs left behind on the sinks and the short curly hairs on the toilet seats. I hope she wears rubber gloves.

In the morning, Gracie stuffs her backpack into a locker, then sits down to study the subway map before we go down for breakfast.

"You globetrotter you, I knew you'd make sense of the subway map. It looks like chicken scratch to me."

"Please, Mother."

I follow her down cement steps into a dingy subway station. "Remember, elbows out." Those are her instructions before we enter a subway car. All the seats are taken so we hang onto a pole, smelling strangers' sour bodies. I'm reading an advertisement for approved latex condoms when she says, "This is our stop. Penn Station." I hold onto her coat tail so we won't get separated. We squeeze out of the door and take the UP escalator. A man in a suit nudges me to one side with his briefcase.

"Mum, I told you. You have to keep to the right."

Outside, my eyes are adjusting to the light. Gracie checks the map and gets her bearings. I tell her there's no way I'd be taking the subway in New York by myself.

"Don't act so helpless. Just because Dad's the boss."

The Macy's store goes on for blocks, with several floors devoted to ladies' wear. I'm thinking, "What more could any woman want?" when Gracie announces, "I'm going to check out the funky little boutiques further down the street. I'll meet you back here at the Starbucks at 11:00."

I wander from one department to the next until I find styles for the mature woman. I buy a camel-coloured blazer, two pairs of dress pants (brown and navy), a white T-shirt with a lacy neckline, and a red cotton blouse. Quite a shopping spree, if you ask me. At 11:00, with a paper cup of coffee in my hand, I rest my aching feet.

When Gracie arrives, I recite, *"Macy's, Macy's, give me your answer do, I'm half crazy all for the love of you."* She rolls her eyes. I pull out my purchases, one by one, to show her.

"Jesus Mother, you hardly went wild and crazy. You could've found this stuff at The Bay."

"Maybe I'm just not a wild and crazy girl. How about you, what did you buy?"

"Nothing."

We stroll along Fifth Avenue arm-in-arm and I start singing "Downtown". I'm no Petula Clark, but I'm downtown and I'm singing.

"Mum, you're embarrassing me." She yanks away her arm and stomps off in a huff. Temper temper.

Across the intersection, I catch up to her. "Let's find a nice place for lunch."

The first restaurant we come to is The Chipotle Mexican Grill. Gracie studies the menu in the window. When she's paying her own way, she checks prices. "Looks okay."

"Is it Chi-poe-tle or Chi-paw-tle?"

"It's Chi-pote-lay, Mum. It's a smoked chili pepper."

"I suppose it's Spanish. You'd know."

To fit through the doorway with my shopping bags, I have to turn sideways. The waiter reminds me of Frankie Avalon in the

Beach Party movies, shiny black hair combed back, wavy. He's muscular and very good looking.

Two menus the size of cookie sheets cover our little table. Planting his feet shoulder-width apart, he announces, "I'm Hor-Hay and I will be your server." I can tell he's nervous. "Today's specials are Po-so-lay soup and Chicken Parmesan and our cocktail special is the Blood Orange Margarita. The appetizer of the day is Creamy Guacamole with toasted tortilla wedges." A white linen napkin is tucked into the waist of his black dress pants and another is draped over his forearm. "May I bring you ladies a beverage?"

"Ice tea please," Gracie says.

"Make that two."

"What did he say his name was?" I ask.

"Hor-hay. It's George in Spanish, Mother. He's Latino. Cuban I bet."

"Is Latino the same as Hispanic?"

"More or less."

So far we're the only customers in the place. "Grand Central Station is grand, isn't it? It made me think back to when I was growing up. Us cousins used to play Canasta at the kitchen table and when we got too rambunctious, my mother would say, 'It's just like Grand Central Station in here', and click her tongue like this."

"How about the luncheon platter for two?" Gracie suggests.

"What is it?"

She points to the menu and reads out loud. "Smoky Chi-pote-lay corn-Jalapeno bread, black bean dip with veggies and tomato salsa."

"As long as it's not too spicy. You decide. You're the one who lived in Mexico."

"Do you always have to bring that up? I suppose you'd like me to order in Spanish, too."

We paid for her to go on an exchange to Mexico after she graduated from grade twelve and that's the thanks I get.

"What do you like best about New York so far, Mum?"

"Besides Macy's you mean? Oh . . . the daffodils in Central Park, the hustle and bustle on the streets, the neon lights. That's how "Downtown" popped into my mind. They always play that song on CJGX. And how about you?"

"Standing on the corner of Time Square last night after the play, the warm spring air, crowds of people, traffic noise, the energy. And in the midst of it all, this big crane with the guy in the bucket peeling off one billboard and pasting on a new one. A bull's eye symbol."

"Are you lovely ladies ready to order?" Faintly visible through Hor-Hay's white shirt is dark chest hair. There are beads of perspiration on his forehead.

Gracie says, "The luncheon platter for two please."

"An excellent choice if I may say so."

"Gracie, do you remember when you won that fridge magnet kit from CBC Radio? I *heart* New York? You must have been about fourteen."

"Yeah. I still have it somewhere, packed away in a box."

We're sipping our ice tea with a slice of lime. I lean over and say in a church whisper, "Take a gander at those two."

A sixty-plus woman in spike heels and a blonde bouffant hairdo sweeps into the café. With her finger in the air, she demands a table for two. Her white wool coat is a tent with a fur fringe around gaping sleeves. Hanging from her arm is a huge red purse. I can feel a gust of wind from her coat as she passes. Through her copper-coloured makeup, you can see large age spots. One side of her face looks swollen. Maybe she had that stuff injected to puff out the wrinkles and it ended up lopsided.

An elderly woman trails behind with shuffling steps. They sit at the very next table. The younger one is facing me — square glasses with white plastic frames, wrinkled eyelids smeared with violet eye shadow, sunken cheeks, and red lipstick bleeding into the crevices above her top lip. Jewels dangle from her sagging earlobes. The older one sloughs off her white mink coat. I can see the lining is tatty. Her perfume is overpowering.

"I'm Hor-Hay and I will be your server. Today's specials are Po-so-lay soup . . ."

The younger one interrupts him to order two Cokes. Sweat is making his white shirt stick to his back.

"Ma, ya gotta drink somethin'."

"I can't Elaine."

"Take a sip of ya Coke. Ya gotta get some sugar into ya. I'm gonna call Uncle Sid to pick us up."

"I've never been so weak."

"Two lunch specials," she says to Hor-Hay, then gets up. "I'll be right back, Ma. Drink ya Coke."

There are stains on the old lady's blouse. She's wearing black ballerina slippers, Tender Tootsies with silver bows, and no panty hose or socks.

"SoHo and NoHo. Do you know what they're short for?" I ask Gracie.

"Yeah. Remember that street we passed H-o-u-s-t-o-n? It's actually pronounced How-ston, not Hew-ston. SoHo is south of Houston and NoHo is north. I would give my eye teeth to live in a bachelor apartment in Manhattan. If I could save up enough rent money for a year, I'd just write and paint, hang out in coffee shops."

A lamebrain notion for a twenty-five-year-old, I think, but I'm careful not to raise my eyebrows. She says these are her salad days, whatever that means. If you ask me, it's about time she settled down. I can't keep count of how many boyfriends she's lived with.

"Elaine, where were you? I've been hangin' onto the table so I don't fall."

"I'm gonna take ya to a hospital. They'll give ya some IV's."

"I need an ambulance. I can't walk."

"An ambulance'll take you to St. Vincent Hospital. You know what happened to Leonard when they took him there."

"I can't walk."

"I'll be right back. I have to go to the bathroom. Drink some Coke."

"I can't drink."

Our meal arrives, arranged like a work of art, so I take a picture of the platter, of the wedges of bread standing up.

Gracie says, "Have you noticed people say M'nhattan rather than Man-hattan?"

"And f'ntastic. How many times did Abigail say f'ntastic in that play?"

"Do you like the lunch, Mum?"

"Sure. I'll pass on the salsa, though. Too hot for my taste."

The old lady closes her eyes and leans further and further to one side. I reach out because she's about to topple off her chair. The daughter returns from God-knows-where, all worked up.

"Where were ya, Elaine?"

"I was talking to Uncle Abe. He can't come. I'm gonna call a taxi."

"I can't walk to a taxi."

"It was that attorney upstairs. When he talked to ya about the divorce papers, he got y'all upset. Eat some chicken. You'll feel betta."

"I can't eat, I said."

Gracie and I can see two policemen standing outside on the corner of West 34th St and 5th Ave. We watch Elaine approach them, her sleeves flapping like wings. She leads them into the café and over to her mother slumped in the chair.

"Ma, these cops are gonna help ya walk to the taxi. I'm a nervous wreck."

"Eleanor, how old are you?"

"I was born in 1926."

"Are you in pain?"

"The worst pain ever. I can't walk. I've never been this weak. I don't know what's wrong with me."

One of the policemen turns to Elaine and says, "Lady, she can't walk. We're not going to carry her to the taxi."

"Okay. Okay. Call an ambulance then. Waiter, put this food in take-out containas, would ya? I'll just be a minute, Ma. I gotta make a couple phone calls."

The officers are back on the street corner, talking to each other with hand gestures and laughing.

"May I tempt you ladies with our dessert menu?" Hor-Hay asks us. He lists several cheesecakes, then emphasizes the *Tres Leches* Cake topped with fresh raspberries. You can tell he has memorized his lines. "The secret is the three-milk soaking." The whole time, he's tapping his fingers on the order pad.

"Let's have the cake, Gracie. My treat. Where do you suppose raspberries grow? They must bring them in by truck."

"After lunch, Mum, I want to go to Tiffany's. They have one whole floor for just gold and another floor for silver. Honestly, I'd settle for one of their boxes. They're turquoise with "Tiffany & Co." embossed on the lid."

"Ma, the ambulance is here for ya. They'll give you some IV's."

An ambulance is double-parked outside, yellow lights flashing. A young woman in a uniform comes in, squats down to Eleanor's eye level, and asks, "Eleanor, what's the matter? Where's your pain?" Her voice is very gentle.

"In my back."

"We're going to help you into this wheelchair and take you to the hospital in an ambulance."

"Don't forget my fur coat."

"You're gonna be okay, Eleanor."

We can see Elaine outside with two styrofoam take-out containers in one hand and her big red purse in the other. Eleanor is being wheeled up a ramp into the ambulance, her worn mink coat draped over her shoulders. They've taken off her wig. She has dabs of grey hair pasted to her scalp. I reach into my purse for my camera, walk over to the window, and take a picture. I see Hor-Hay out there leaning against the wall with one knee up, puffing on a cigarette while they load Eleanor. When I turn away from the window, I can feel two burning spots on my back.

"Eleanor and Elaine, we'll have a picture to remember them."
I put my camera away. "I bet they used to be beautiful, wear
expensive clothes, have men come calling, probably even shop at
Tiffany's, but not anymore." Well, you should have seen the look
on Gracie's face.

"I can't believe you took a picture of them. How would you
like someone taking your picture while you're being loaded into
an ambulance with your wig off?"

"You don't need to be so crabby. They'll never see the picture."
I can feel my neck go red and blotchy.

"You're the one who goes to church, then you make fun of a
sick old woman. I suppose you'll show the picture to Auntie Bea
and tell her all about these two Manhattan babes, like it was a
Broadway play?"

"Gracie, keep your voice down."

Hor-Hay is heading our way with a black folder in his hand.
He's antsy, fidgets with our bill. I can smell cigarette smoke. His
manner has changed. "You can pay at the bar," he says abruptly.

We've lost interest in our dessert by this time. Soggy cake in
red puddles. A few lunchtime stragglers, all women, lean forward
talking at their tables. Gracie won't look at me. She stares at a boy
clearing tables. If she could go to her room and slam the door, she
would.

I say, "I don't want to lug all these parcels along to the MOMA,
never mind *The Lion King*. Let's take them back to the hostel."

"Fine." Gracie stands up and wraps her coral Pashmina scarf
from Chinatown around the collar of her new black jacket. She
puts some cash, her share, into the folder, then heads for the door.

"I'll leave the tip." After mentally calculating my half of the lunch plus the two desserts, then adding 10%, I walk over to the bar, leave the folder and say, "Thank you". I'm doing up my coat buttons when Hor-Hay slaps the vinyl folder with the back of his hand. "You call this a tip?" he says, and screws up his face. The other customers must've heard him. He was quite loud. Of all the nerve! He should be thankful he's got a job. My ears are on fire.

Gracie is looking at some posters in the entrance. This part is hard to believe . . . she turns around and marches right up to Hor-Hay, her nose so close to his mouth that she must be able to smell his breath. He leans back, and does she let . . . him . . .have . . . it . . . in Spanish. She spits out, "*Blankety-blank intimidate blankety-blank maa-drey!*" Boy is she hot under the collar! Then she grabs my sleeve and spins me around. She points to a sign at the door and reads it out loud. "Dine with us. Empire State Building Chi-pote-lay Mexican Grill. Mum, this is the Empire State Building. We just had lunch in the Empire State Building and didn't even know it."

Off we go. She's laughing. I'm a little shaken.

Down Below

A WHITE BELLYBUTTON. THAT'S WHAT I'M thinking, my index finger pressing the indented doorbell, lumpy and bumpy with years of fresh paint. Peony blossoms the colour of red wine are heavy on bushes flanking the steps. White wicker chairs and a low table have been arranged in a cluster to invite conversation on the wraparound porch. Above my head, a hanging basket bursts with coral geraniums, English ivy, and a sprinkling of bacopa. I can hear the buzz of the doorbell. A short bald man with smiling dentures opens the door and extends his hand in greeting. "You must be Grace."

"Yes." I step over the threshold onto a jute floormat and set down my overnight bag. "I made a reservation online." My bones are aching after a set-to with Geoff and five night shifts in a row. I feel like crawling into a hole and staying there.

He must have rehearsed that smile. "The Barnum and Bailey Room. I'm Don. My wife will tell you I belong in her antique collection. *Har. Har.*" Don looks dapper in his white golf shirt with narrow navy and green horizontal stripes, and his khaki pants with a crease. I wish he would back up a little. He's too close and too smiley for my liking.

"Pleased to meet you." I slip off my Birkenstocks without bending over, line them up against the wall. The oak hardwood has a high gloss finish. Geoff is convinced that you can't tell the difference between our laminate flooring and real oak.

"It's your first time staying with us?" Don's eyes are warbled by the lenses in his glasses.

"It is."

"May I ask what brings you to our fair city?"

"Just passing through on my way to Kelowna. Actually, I grew up here."

"Did you?" He furrows his brow and rubs his scalp. Flakes of dandruff settle on his golf shirt, just above the pocket bulging with a pack of cigarettes.

"May I ask what you do for a living?"

"I'm a nurse."

"Ahh, a lady with a lamp."

I pick up my Air Canada tote bag.

"The Barnum and Bailey Room is one floor up. Do you need help with your luggage?"

"No thank you, I just have this one." I set my foot on the first step.

"We serve breakfast between 7:30 and 9:00. What time would you prefer?"

"Eight o'clock please. I want to be on the road by 9:00."

I've reached a landing partway up the long flight of stairs and am catching my breath.

"On the bedside table, you'll find a breakfast menu. Just fill it out and slip it under the door. Keys are in the lock — one for your room, the other for the front door."

I look back down at him. "Okay." He is resting one hand on the knob of the ornate newel post at the base of the stairs and gesturing with the other.

I turn and climb the second set of stairs. I must be out of his view. He calls after me. "If you would like us to recommend a restaurant or if there's anything else me or my wife can do to make your stay more pleasant, just let us know."

I have escaped Dapper Don, who no doubt earned a framed diploma for successfully completing a two-day Hospitality Training course.

There are four doors, two on either side of the hall, each with a brass nameplate. I open the door labelled "Barnum and Bailey" and find myself at the circus — all reds and yellows, posters of performing geese and a musical donkey. I close the door behind me. After I pee, I sprinkle a little talc on my inner thighs, chafed after a full day in the car, then flop down on the bed with my head on a calliope pillow sham. The mattress is comfy. My back is aching and my legs are swollen. I close my eyes to shut out the busy wallpaper. The house is perfectly quiet. My breathing slows.

Shiftwork will be the death of me. Geoff has no clue what it's like.

The Maple Leafs won, I had given in to oral sex, I thought it was the opportune moment.

His response was, "It wouldn't make any sense. Finances . . . mortgage . . . retirement planning . . . logical . . . blah, blah, blah."

"I could take out a student loan."

" . . . loss of income . . . benefits . . . long-term financial projection . . . impractical. . . never earn back . . . stock market . . ."

He peppered me with questions he knew I wouldn't be able to answer. "Have you calculated . . . ? How much have you got in your pension plan?"

He didn't raise his voice, he didn't have to.

It ended the way it always ends, with me dissolving into tears.

I've never told him I wanted to have a baby. We were twenty when we agreed not to have children. How could I have known I'd change my mind? Now it's too late.

On the edge of dozing off, it comes to me. I sit bolt upright on my bedspread featuring clowns with white faces and huge red mouths. Dapper Don. I felt a gust of cold air when he shook my hand. Like when Geoff told me it was time I lost some weight. "A lot of weight." It was affecting his libido.

He's not Don. He's Mr. Johnson, my creepy grade eight teacher and principal of Sir Wilfrid Laurier School. I can hardly believe it. I'm in Mr. Johnson's house. I've been ambushed.

A yellow Hilroy scribbler with name-nom *Grace Schmidt* and subject-sujet *Social Studies* on the front cover, I can see it.

My pencil, my eraser, and my Parker pen with the peacock blue cartridge resting in the little ditch at the top of my sloped wooden desk, I can see that, too. It's my last year in public school. After grade eight graduation, I'll move up to high school, like flying up from Brownies to Girl Guides. My brother says there isn't any recess in high school and that if you get in trouble for not having your homework done or for talking back, the teacher can give you detention. Writing in textbooks isn't allowed because you have to turn them in at the end of the year. Not that I get in trouble or write in my books anyway.

In September, I took a silent self-imposed vow of neatness in the hopes that my teacher might choose one of my scribblers for the Notebook Competition at The Fair. The proper name is The Agricultural Exhibition, but everyone calls it The Fair.

Sometimes when I use my pink-and-blue eraser to rub out a mistake, I accidentally make a little hole in the paper. I tear out the page and recopy it at home after supper. *A sunbeam, a sunbeam, Jesus wants me for a sunbeam to shine for Him each day.*

Mr. Johnson is pacing up and down the aisles, making sure we're taking notes. "Boys and girls, today we are studying India. The population of India is one billion. The official language is Hindi. H-i-n-d-i. Write that down." He has this habit of stopping, rising up on his tippy toes, staying there for a few seconds, then back down onto his heels. He probably wishes he was taller.

"The religion in India is Hindu. That's H-i-n-d-u. New Dell-High is the capital city. D-e-l-h-i." He uses a wooden pointer to show us the location of New Dell-High on the map that pulls down at the front, then carries on. "People eat mostly fish curry and rice." Pause. "Cricket and field hockey are the most popular sports."

This is Mr. Johnson's first year at our school. He is the principal and my first man teacher. We heard he's a really good ball player and that he just got married.

"I have a map for each of you." We file past his desk, one row at a time, and take a mimeographed map of India. The first thing we're supposed to do is write our name in the upper right hand corner, then put dots for Calcutta and New Delhi, label the Arabian Sea, the Bay of Bengal, and the Indian Ocean, then colour the map.

I outline India in red, then lean my Laurentian pencil crayon at an angle, using the side of the lead instead of the point. My India is pink. I colour the oceans pastel blue, naturally. In grade six and seven, I won ribbons in the Map Competition at The Fair.

Steve is always getting out of his desk and going to the pencil sharpener at the back. He can never sit still.

The bell goes at four o'clock. Cindy collects our maps for the teacher. Dad will be waiting for me outside in the car. *I try to do my best at home, at school, at play.*

There are twenty-six pupils in grade eight. The girls are taller than the boys. The boys' voices are changing, which is hilarious. Our desks were meant for little kids. They have lids that lift up, with a storage compartment underneath. Mine is in the middle of the classroom. We stay in the same spot for the whole year unless people are fooling around. If that happens, the teacher moves them.

After morning announcements over the intercom, Mr. Johnson says, "Class. Does everyone have their Health textbooks out? Blaine, distribute the notebooks." We had to hand them in yesterday so Mr. Johnson could check them. At the bottom of my last page, he wrote "Good" in red ink.

A chart of Students' Responsibilities is posted on the wall. It's plain, no border of zoo animals in a parade like in younger grades. Along the left side of the chart, in red felt pen, our first names are printed in alphabetical order. Grace S. comes before Steve P. In black, along the top, are our weekly chores. Collect assignments. Blackboard monitor. Garbage. Tidy classroom. Distribute books.

Mr. Johnson is waiting for us to settle down. He always wears a suit jacket, grey pants, a white shirt, tie, and polished shoes. Today his tie has diagonal stripes, blue and navy. Queen Elizabeth is above his head. Exactly the same picture in the same black frame hangs above the blackboard in every classroom. We always sing *God Save the Queen* at school assemblies. *O Canada* at the beginning and *God Save the Queen* at the end.

There are tall windows all the way up to the ceiling on one wall, with a view of the ball diamond, houses across the street, and the sky. On the other side are posters — The Golden Rule, Every Good Boy Deserves Fudge, ROYGBIV, Man Very Early Made Jars Stand Up Nearly Perpendicular, Play by the rules, Good jobs await high school graduates.

Social Studies is after recess. "Turn to Chapter Five on Pakistan. Are you ready to take dictation? In high school, you will be expected to take dictation." Pause. "English is the official language of Pakistan. Write that down." Pause. "Maw-zlum is the religion. M-o-s-l-e-m."

"Okay, who can tell me the religion in India?"

Cindy's hand shoots up. She calls him "Mr. Pick-it-and-Flick-it" behind his back because he does just that.

"Cindy."

"The religion in India is Hindu." We're supposed to answer questions in complete sentences.

"That's correct."

The letter *H* for Hindu + *I* for India = *H.I.* I'll use the letters in the alphabet to help memorize for my tests. The letter *M* for Moslem + *P* for Pakistan = *M.P.*

"Any questions?"

I put up my hand.

"Grace."

"Is New Dell-High the same as New Dellee?" My father always makes us keep quiet during the CBC radio news at dinnertime and I heard the announcer saying something about New Dellee.

"No."

Even after he says "No", he keeps staring at me like I did something wrong. Then he leafs through the pages in his textbook kinda rough. My stomach starts to ache.

"The capital city of Pakistan is Karachi. Make sure you spell it right. K-a-r-a-c-h-i."

It's a Thursday in the middle of June, the day the kitten falls down the outhouse. I'm wearing my new pop-top with navy sailboats and red-and-white lifesavers, and my white pedal pushers with a twisty rope for a belt. When I come home for dinner, Fluffy is meowing like crazy. She's a tabby cat with the tips of her ears frozen off. When I'm leaving, she almost trips me on the steps, then cuts in front of me on the sidewalk. I stoop down to pet her. Usually she purrs and arches her back, but this time she meows even louder, dashes off, then comes back and goes around and around my ankles in circles. *Pussy cat, pussy cat, where have you been?* She bolts, then comes back yowling. The black slits in her yellow eyes are bulging like some evil creature. She must be sick.

My father is in the car listening to the CBC farm report. His hairy arm, powdered with grain dust, pokes out of the open window, elbow first. There's an untanned white band under his wristwatch.

"Dad, there's something wrong with the cat."

"Get in, Gracie. It's just a barn cat."

"But Dad, she's trying to tell me something."

"It's quarter to one. You'll be late for school."

Fluffy disappears through an opening under the carragana hedge. I follow her in the direction of the outhouse. The door is open and the lid of the little hole is up. She springs onto the plywood seat and pokes her button nose down into the hole and bawls. I peer into the hole. I can't see anything, but I can hear a puny little squeak from below. I run back to the car.

"Dad, Dad, a kitten fell down the outhouse."

"What am I supposed to do about it?" He's getting mad.

"You've gotta help please Daddy please."

"You're gonna be late."

"I won't get in trouble if you write me a note."

"It's just a stupid cat."

"Please."

"There's a truckload of barley I have to get into the granary. Look at that dark cloud in the west." He turns off the key in the ignition, the radio goes silent, he gets out of the car. I hear him mumble "For Christ's sake" under his breath.

I fetch a flashlight from the garage, like he tells me, then catch up with him. The outhouse is the place where he reads *The Western Producer* after supper even though we have a flush toilet in the house. I never set foot in there because of the stink. He shines the flashlight down into the hole and we both see a little ball of fur squealing non-stop. It's brown and blends in with the crap. Fluffy is hysterical.

"Get a *maltj* pail from the icehouse."

I run to the little yellow building which doesn't have ice in it anymore. Dad is holding a long piece of rope. He ties one end to the handle of the pail with a bulky knot. He hands me the flashlight.

I can smell onions on his breath. We eat our big meal at noon. Liver and onions today. I hate liver, so I just ate the mashed potatoes and carrots, and lime Jello with whipped cream. Dad raises cattle, pigs, and chickens, and Mum cooks all of the parts — the liver and kidneys, even the chicken gizzards. My heart is beating fast. It's hard to believe my father is rescuing a kitten. I know he drowns newborn kittens, even though I've never caught him in the act. Our barn cats mysteriously have only one kitten every spring except for that time I was the first one to discover the litter of seven under the granary.

Hand over hand, he lowers the galvanized pail down the big hole. I keep the flashlight shining on the kitten. Whenever I forget to breathe through my mouth, I smell a mixture of poop and mothballs. There are brown splatters on the walls, and turds are all smushed together in a heap with two peaks. The kitten won't crawl into the pail even after Dad tilts it. It's a furball paralyzed on a wad of streaked toilet paper.

"*Dumma Katze.*" He yanks the pail up by the rope and huffs. "I tried, girlie. I have to get that load of barley into the granary before it rains."

"But Dad . . ."

Fluffy weaves in and out of our legs, screeching non-stop.

"We have to think of some other way."

"I've got one more idea and that's it," he says. "I've wasted enough time."

He walks over to the machine-shed and brings back a long board. He pushes it down the big hole. I have to use both hands to hold the flashlight because they're shaking. I know this is the kitten's last chance. I don't care about the stink anymore. Dad leans the board at an angle, lets go of it, and straightens up. My face is level with the seat and so is Fluffy's. She meows instructions to her kitten. It stretches out one front paw and sets it down on the board. Then the other front paw. The kitten clings onto the board with its einsy-weinsy claws and creeps up, halting now and then, cheered on by its mother. I let out a little squeal. I'm not sure if my father is following the kitten's progress, but the rough denim of his overalls brushes against my arm. Close-up I see a metal rivet where the pocket is attached to his pantleg.

When the putrid shivering kitten has almost reached us, Dad pins Fluffy in place with a grimy leather work glove. She growls a low throaty rumble. With his free hand, he plucks the shitty kitten from the board and plunks it onto the lid of the little hole.

"Fill this pail with soapy water and get some rags."

I scrub the kitten on the grass. It twists, hisses, and scratches my arms. When I set it free, Fluffy sinks her teeth into its loose neck skin, carries it to a sunny patch on the sidewalk, and licks it dry. I can hear her coo and scold while I put away the pail and rags. *All things bright and beautiful, all creatures great and small, all things wise and wonderful, the Lord God made them all.* I have yet to notice the stains on my new white pedal pushers with a twisty rope for a belt.

The kitten doesn't matter to Dad. As far as he is concerned, the only reason to have cats on a farm is to keep the mouse population under control. He must've hosed off the board and put it back in the machine-shed. Across the yard, a hydraulic lift raises the box of the truck to dump barley into the grain auger. The auger makes a big racket. I can't see Dad in the cloud of chaff.

Mum will have finished the dishes and will be vacuuming or dusting. She doesn't like cats, refuses to allow them in the house. What happened won't matter to her. What will matter are the stains on my pedal-pushers: *Cleanliness is next to Godliness.*

I put Dad's note on Mr. Johnson's desk on Friday morning. "Gracie had to help with farm work on Thursday afternoon." Little do I know what he has in store for me.

We only have a few pages left in our Science textbook, about how flowers reproduce, then the chapter reviews. Mr. Johnson is standing very close, facing the side of my desk. Too close. I smell Aqua Velva. He says to the class, "Some flowers have both male and female parts. Others are either male or female. The female organ of a flower is called the pistil. P-i-s-t-i-l. Settle down, boys. The male organ is called the stamen. S-t-a-m-e-n. You'll see a diagram on page 124. Class, pay attention to where the stamen and the pistil are, so you can label them on your diagram." I keep my eyes on my textbook. He hasn't moved.

He rises up on his toes, leans forward, then lowers his heels, resting a clump of grey flannel on my desk. Mr. Johnson's personal stamen is no more than eight inches away from my hand as I write "pistil — female" in peacock blue ink in my Science scribbler. Then, on the next line, "stamen — male." I keep my head down. I can see *it* out of the corner of my eye.

"On your final exam, you'll be expected to label the diagrams correctly." Pause. "The colourful parts of the flower are called the petals. He enunciates the letter *t* in petals. The petals combine to make up the ... ?" Pause.

He rises up on his toes again and *it* slides off my desk. He turns, lowers himself onto his heels, and walks to the front of the class. Susan N. raises her hand and Mr. Johnson nods.

"The petals combine to make up the corolla."

"Correct."

"Come up to the front and get your diagram of the flower. Beginning with this row, in orderly fashion."

We learned about the eye and ear in Health, but not the rest of the human body. Mum calls a girl's private parts her "B.O." (short for Body Odour). When I'm taking a bath, she reminds me to wash my B.O. My brother told me that a boy's thing is called a dinky. I looked up the word in my Webster's New World Dictionary, but it isn't there. After Dad and the hired man castrated calves, they were washing up on the back step before supper and I heard them talking about balls. So it must've been the principal's dinky and balls that were plopped on my desk.

Being short is an advantage for Mr. Johnson. He can stand next to me, rise onto his toes while we write down the parts of a flower because the question might be on our exam, then lower his private parts onto my desk.

When I corrected his pronunciation of New Delhi, he could've made me write one hundred lines: "I will not correct the principal in front of the class." There's no such thing as detention in public school, but he could've called me over the intercom. "Grace Schmidt, report to the principal's office when the noon hour bell rings." He could've taken away my recesses for a week.

He could've made me apologize. He could've even given me the strap. But when you have a smart aleck on your hands, you have to show her who's boss and make sure she won't blab.

It's report card day. Just before the bell goes, Mr. Johnson gives each of us a big brown envelope with our name typed on the outside. I open mine on the front seat of the car while Dad is driving. Sure enough, I got all A's and A+'s, but under Teacher's Comments, it says: "Grace is a promising student, but needs to improve her attitude." There's Mr. Johnson's signature on a line with "D. Johnson" typed below. I look down at my white canvas runners. I will have some explaining to do.

I wake up in Mr. Johnson's house. My first conscious thought is: *I'm sick of being married.* My second thought is: *It's time Mr. Johnson faced up to his past.* At breakfast, I'll tell him I'd like to have a word with him in private. He'll probably take me into an office. I'll look him straight in the eye and say, "You're not Don to me, you're Mr. Johnson." He'll still be smiling at this point. "Do you know what I remember about grade eight, Mr. Johnson? When I was a naive thirteen-year-old? What I remember is you resting your genitals on my desk. You hazed me. I've told my 'Mr. Johnson's Testicles' story at parties — it always brings a laugh. But let's scrutinize your behaviour through mature eyes. You abused your power, Mr. Johnson. You deserved to be fired and blacklisted. Never to teach again." He'll deny it, of course, try to leave, but I won't let up. "You knew I'd be too afraid to tell." I'll increase the volume. "But I'm not afraid of you anymore, Mr. Johnson." He'll try to hush me. "I couldn't care less who hears me. Will your wife believe *me*? Or you?"

I descend the stairs armed with resolve and join five strangers around a lavish breakfast table. It's a tight squeeze for me to fit into chairs with arms. "So round, so firm, so fully packed," that's what Dad would say if he were alive. At each place is a clear glass bowl of yogurt sprinkled with granola and garnished with a fresh gooseberry. We introduce ourselves while Mr. Johnson fills our coffee cups. An elderly woman says, "I'm in the city for my second round of chemo." Two other women, one at either end, are touring BC. Most likely Lesbians. Lesbians tend to gravitate toward B & Bs. Facing me is a fresh-faced couple on their honeymoon.

Mr. Johnson stands behind my chair and pushes a dog-eared black-and-white class picture in my line of vision. There I am, standing on a wooden bench, sandwiched between Steve Polachuk and Cindy Hess. I was chubby already. My mother rolled my bangs under with one curler the night before. There he is, standing on the floor at the far right. Mr. Johnson.

"You said this was your home town. It took me a while, but then I remembered you. Little Gracie Schmidt. Did you know I was principal of Sir Wilfrid Laurier at twenty- two?"

Nerves prompt me to say: "Oh, grade eight. That's when I learned about the birds and the bees." I say it cheerfully enough. " . . . the birds and the bees," but my audible swallow at the end might give me away. That is, if Mr. Johnson remembers. He laughs at my remark and passes the photo around. "Grace is the blonde girl in the back row, second from the left." Other guests contribute anecdotes from their own coming-of-age repertoire.

Dad must have demanded an explanation for the Teacher's Comments on my report card. How could I have told him that Mr. Johnson rested his private parts on my desk eight inches away from my right hand just as I was about to print in my Hilroy scribbler? With my cartridge pen in peacock blue ink. There's no way I could have told either of my parents. Mum turned off the TV if there was any kissing, and refused to allow Hallowe'en costumes with tails. No kissing, no tails, and certainly no talk of what's down below. How could I have told her?

We can hear bustling in the kitchen while Mr. Johnson, now seated at the head of the table with a mug of coffee in hand, recaps his career as an educator, boasts about having been promoted to Superintendent of Schools in his thirties and having retired early with an ample pension. This is his second marriage, he volunteers, then lowers his voice to confide. "The B & B was my wife's idea. She's much younger than me, you know. It gives her a little something to do."

It must be the same performance every morning with a new audience. Or is it for my benefit?

Mr. Johnson raises his chin and turns his gaze to acknowledge the entrance of Mrs. Johnson the Second, bearing plates of turkey bacon and French toast powdered with icing sugar. She's younger than me and, as my father would say, has kept her girlish figure. Mr. Johnson introduces her as Giselle, prompting the table talk to swing over to Quebec and how Canada is more culturally rich than the USA thanks to bilingualism and biculturalism. What a paragon of enlightenment we profess to be.

We've finished our breakfast. I'll wait until the others excuse themselves before I approach Mr. Johnson. I'm still hungry. There'll probably be a Timmy's drive-through on the way out of town. The Lesbians dilly-dally, unfolding a map on the table and plotting their route, so I go to my room to get my bag.

Back upstairs at the circus, I brush my teeth and zip up my toiletry bag. When I pay my bill, that's when I'll say, "Mr. Johnson,

I remember the time you rested your sticky genitals on my desk to punish me for correcting you in class." He'll be indignant, say how dare I accuse him of such a thing, and in his own home no less. I'll put on my shoes, grab my bag, and make a quick exit.

My bill is on a little side table with brochures at the door. Mr. Johnson appears. I pay in cash so he can't track me down.

"I hope you've enjoyed your stay and that you'll be back soon, Grace." The dazzling dentures again. "Drive carefully."

Here's my opening. My mouth is dry, my cheeks are flushed, I fumble with my wallet, slide my feet into my Birkenstocks, and say, "Thank you."

The only two words that come out of my mouth are, "Thank you."

I'm in my car heading east on the Number 1, thinking about the day the kitten fell down the outhouse. I named it Kissy. During harvest, when our neighbour was hauling grain to the elevator, he ran over it with his truck.

Chicken

Box 98
Kedleston, SK
Feb. 10, 1990

Dear Stewart,

Harvey Sinclair Woods. It's been years since I've seen that name in print. Thank you for sending me a copy of your father's obituary. It was a surprise to learn that my name was in his address book. Mind you, I haven't moved since the thirties.

Did you know that Harvey courted me before he married your mother? On Saturdays after the hardware store closed, he would change into a fresh shirt, slick back his hair with pomade, and come calling in a horse-drawn buggy (or sleigh in winter). I'd serve him tea with home-baked cookies in the sitting room. I had been taught that the way to a man's heart was through his stomach, which didn't prove true in this case. My mother never let us out of her sight. Harvey had the gift of the gab and I, like any good listener, had plenty of questions. He would expound on his personal ambitions and on his passion, namely horses.

I fully expected him to propose, but he stopped coming around. In time I learned he was bestowing his favours upon Dorothy Heston, who was prettier than me and had a more abundant dowry. I was heartbroken, as only a nineteen-year-old can be. Harvey and Dorothy's wedding photo appeared in *The Kedleston Times*. In the write-up, it said they would be relocating to Swift Current where Harvey had accepted a position at a larger hardware store.

I never got over him. He was the only suitor who made my heart flutter. Resigned to my destiny as an old maid, I went to Normal School in Regina, then returned home to teach. Latin became my passion. I retired after forty-five years and live in my childhood home with no one calling on Saturday evenings.

You can be proud of your father's litany of achievements and your parents' long marriage. They were blessed to have had a son.

Absit iniuria verbis. Let injury be absent from these words.

Miss Myrtle Cole

P.S. I notice as I address this envelope that you are a university professor. My life must seem small in comparison with yours.

———

Stewart Woods:

You said my name was in his address book. What the Hell was it doing there? I paid back the measly $12.00 he loaned me in the dirty thirties when we were going through tough times. My daughter Marlene came down with pneumonia, she was 9 years old. Doc Wright said she had to be in the hospital under a steam tent and I didn't have no money. It was before the CCF brought in hospitalization. The bank turned me down for a loan, bastards said I didn't have no collateral. The wife was crying her eyes out, we thought our girl was going to die, I had to come up with the money. So I went to the Marshall-Wells and asked Harvey for a loan. He was the manager. I paid it back as soon as I sold my wheat that fall. It must've been twenty-five years later I went with a Farmers Union delegation to Regina to protest the increase in the tax on fuel. Harvey was the Minister of Highways. I can still see him in that posh office sitting behind a desk in a three-piece suit with his starched shirt collar and his engraved cufflinks. Our spokesman presented our case and Harvey leaned back in his fancy chair and said he couldn't do nothing for us. He singled me out and said he was confident his old friend Mr. Hryniuk would understand there's a limit to the money in the government coffers. It was a personal dig and I never forgave him. In the next election campaign, Ross Thatcher introduced purple gas for farmers. I guess they found money in the government coffers when they wanted to get re-elected.

George Hryniuk

———

Box 146
Vanguard, Sask. S5H 8C9
Feb. 15, 1990

Stewart,

I didn't know Harv passed away until your letter came in the mail. It puts me in mind of that old song, *Gonna Take a Sentimental Journey*.

We worked together at the Marshall-Wells for close to thirty years. Other employees came and went. Younger fellows vied for positions in bigger places. Girls had to quit when they got married. But the two of us were the constants. Middle of the morning and middle of the afternoon, we sat on packing boxes in the storeroom for our coffee breaks and chewed the fat about politics, taxes, crops, the price of nails, the higher-ups in head office and their lamebrain ideas, and of course the weather. Harv drank Maxwell House instant coffee with Carnation evaporated milk. He knew the batting averages of all the Yankees and he was horse crazy, could tell you who won the Preakness and the Kentucky Derby, the owners' names, how much jockeys weighed.

Harv was an up-and-comer, that was obvious as soon as he arrived in Swift Current. Not like me, I'm the type who's satisfied with a steady paycheck and less responsibility, what they call stress today. He worked his way up from clerk to lumber supervisor to manager. He built a brand new house and took your mother on some nice trips. I remember him passing cigars around when you were born and bringing in the program from your university graduation, pointing out your name with letters after it.

After he was elected MLA in '64, we kinda lost touch. When I retired, we moved to Vanguard so my wife could look after her parents. I don't keep up with the Swift Current news.

Harv was a decent hardworking man. I looked up to him. Don't pay any attention to rumours. Some guys were jealous because he made something of himself.

Yours truly,
John Wiens

———

GRAND LODGE OF ANCIENT FREE AND
ACCEPTED MASONS OF CANADA
IN THE PROVINCE OF SASKATCHEWAN

#19 – 3948 Albert St. S
Regina, SK
Feb. 24, 1990

To the family of Master Mason Harvey Woods:

The Brotherhood of Freemasonry mourns the passing of Master Mason Harvey Woods. He was an exemplary brother, having attained the Order's third degree. As a plural affiliate, he maintained his membership with both the Regina Lodge and the Tampa Bay Florida Lodge and was named a lifetime member of the Swift Current Lodge, where he received his first degree.

Freemasonry provides an opportunity for men to meet and enjoy friendly companionship. It is the oldest and largest world-wide fraternity dedicated to the Brotherhood of Man under the Fatherhood of a Supreme

Being. Brothers are guided by strict moral principles. Self-improvement and goodwill toward all mankind are promoted. Master Mason Woods practised the principles of brotherly love, charity, and truth in his daily life.

On behalf of The Grand Lodge of Free and Accepted Masons of Canada in the Province of Saskatchewan, I extend sympathy to you and your family.

G. Thorson, for David S. Fitchner, Grand Master

———

Feb. 21, 1990

Just seeing that name Woods on an envelope addressed to my deceased mother got me fired up. Harvey Woods used to "have coffee" with my mother when my Dad was at work. I'd come home from school and he'd offer me Life Savers. She'd have lipstick on, and her cheeks would be flushed. Once he was tickling her under her arms, and she shooed me outside, said her and Mr. Woods had some Sunday School business to take care of. I hear he had a boyfriend in Regina after he retired. Maybe he swung both ways. Do me a favour, would you? Take an Exacto knife, cut my mother's name out of his address book, and light a match to it?

Barry Anderson

———

Ste. 768 Greystone Heights
Saskatoon, SK
S0K 9E8
Feb. 27, 1990

Dear Stewart,

It was thoughtful of you to remember your old aunt. I was informed of Harvey's passing by Rachel, but I was interested in reading his obituary.

Of all of my sisters, I was closest to Dorothy. We exchanged letters and pictures and she never missed my birthday.

When Harvey first started calling on her, she thought she had a big fish on the line. I had my reservations because he had jilted a girl named Myrtle Cole. Mother and Dad put on a nice wedding. I was maid-of-honour. (You've seen the pictures — Marcelled hair, shoulder pads and all.) In short order, they moved to Swift Current. I knew he'd lure Dorothy to a bigger place where he could have her all to himself.

Her letters and phone calls were cheery and upbeat, but she missed the family get-togethers. She must've been lonely in Swift Current (and later in Regina), but wouldn't admit it.

I hear you're a professor. Your mother would be very proud of you. Do call if you're ever in Saskatoon. There are some subjects best discussed over a cup of strong tea and slice of my raisin pie.

Your Aunt Madelon

———

First Presbyterian Church
1200 E. Trailview Place
Victoria, BC
V7T 8EO
March 1, 1990

Dear Stewart,

May I extend sympathy on the death of your father from myself and my wife Ruth.

Your letter prompted me to review my eleven years at Calvin Presbyterian Church in Swift Current. Harvey was chairman of the Board and applied his business acumen to the church's finances. Those were the glory days when the pews were more or less filled and a minister was appreciated.

Thank you for the copy of Harvey's obituary. May God comfort you in your time of grief.

Yours in Christ,
Rev. Ian McNeil

———

OFFICE OF THE LIEUTENANT GOVERNOR
GOVERNMENT HOUSE
4607 Dewdney Avenue
Regina, Saskatchewan
S4T 5S0
March 18, 1990

Harvey Sinclair Woods had a distinguished career as a politician and business man spanning five decades. He was a Liberal Member of the Legislative Assembly for

Swift Current from 1964-1970, serving as Minister of Highways for three of those years.

He rose to extraordinary heights in public life, but never wavered from his prairie roots. He exemplified the fundamental spirit of Saskatchewan, serving others.

On behalf of the Legislative Assembly and the people of Saskatchewan, I extend my condolences to the Woods family. Although he will be greatly missed, his proud legacy will live on.

Dr. Sylvia O. Fedoruk
Lieutenant Governor of Saskatchewan

———

#8 Keys Plaza
1450 Palms Drive
Tampa Bay, FL 9172
Feb. 20, 1990

Stewart:

Thank you for the copy of your father's obituary. Harv and I were friends for sixteen years. We used to go to the racetrack when he wintered in Tampa Bay, and in 1984 we travelled to India with a tour group.

America has many old goats,
They send them on bus tours, not boats.

I held your father in high regard and I was saddened to hear of his passing.

With sympathy,
Karl J. Werner

———

Ste. 768 Greystone Heights
Saskatoon, SK
S0K 9E8
March 27, 1990

Dear Stewart,

I'm sorry to have missed you when you were in Saskatoon at a conference. I was in Edmonton with Cheryl during her chemo.

I dreamt about your father the other night. I will try to put on paper what I intended to say to you in person. When one reaches my age, one can't afford to put things off.

I used to get a niggling feeling whenever I was in Harvey's company. You remember Mike and Rachel's 25th when Bill Johnson gave him a push for fondling his wife and it turned into a donnybrook out behind the Legion? They're still talking about it to this day. Faithful Dorothy stood by him, but he never showed his face in Kedleston again. Us ladies called him "Grab-your-ass-Harv" and avoided dancing with him. He tried to grope a couple of the men, but they handled him with their fists, called him "Woody Woodpecker". I'm mad as Hell at him for shaming your mother in front of her own people. And I can only imagine what went on in Swift Current and Regina.

On another subject, Dorothy confided in me about the baby you fathered in high school. He must be in his thirties by now. I hope you've been man enough to own up to your responsibilities.

I better leave this letter on the cupboard for a few days before I mail it in case I get cold feet.

Aunt Madelon

———

First Presbyterian Church
1200 E. Trailview Place
Victoria, BC
V7T 8EO
April 2, 1990

Dear Stewart:

My first letter was not entirely truthful. Although I hesitate to recount unpleasant events when you are grieving, I assume you would want to know the facts. Sufficient time has passed for me to be objective.

In 1967, the congregation of Calvin Presbyterian Church split. This is what prompted your parents' move to Regina. It all started when the Synod introduced a more contemporary Sunday School curriculum. It was inter-active — stories, discussion, crafts, activities — Christian lessons in a secular package. The Board thought the congregation should be consulted, so a meeting was called on a Sunday morning right after the worship service. Harvey chaired the meeting. Mrs. Yackel, the Sunday School Superintendent, outlined the old and new curricula, carefully avoiding any bias. Congregants voiced their opinions primarily along age lines. Older members touted the value of Bible stories and memorization of Scripture verses. Young parents favoured the newer approach. It was a stalemate. I expected Harvey to call for a show of hands or leave it up to the Board to make the final decision. Instead he took the side of the new curriculum, highlighting lessons about respect and bullying. In a booming voice, he declared, "Children have to learn right from wrong." It was the tipping point in the debate. That is until a red-faced young father named Vernon Murdoch stood up and pointed his finger at Harvey. He called him a hypocrite, accusing him of touching his mother inappropriately when she used to be the organist. Harvey sat down. There was a stunned silence, then people started talking among themselves, and left with no decision reached. The following Sunday morning, a Xeroxed statement dotted the pews. Vernon retracted his allegation and apologized for any hurt he may have caused your family.

Your parents sold their house and relocated to Regina where Harvey was serving in the Legislature. Pastoring was next to impossible after the whole kerfuffle. It was the most trying time in my ministry.

Like all of us, Harvey had his strengths and weaknesses. Presbyterians avoid using words such as "fallible" and "errant". We believe that forgiveness cannot be earned, but through the death and resurrection of Christ, our sins are forgiven by the grace of God. It is my prayer that Harvey died without fear or regret and that his soul rests in peace.

Yours in Christ,

Rev. Ian McNeil

———

#8 Keys Plaza
1450 Palms Drive
Tampa Bay, FL 9172
March 10, 1990

Stewart:

There is so much more. Excuse my proclivity for ditties. It was a habit that bugged Harv.

> *Abrakadabra Kalamazoo!*
> *Hinky dinky parlez-vous.*
> *Ask me no questions,*
> *I'll tell you no lies.*
> *KJ and Harv,*
> *the suspense, the surprise.*

Harv was a customer at my outdoor gear store in Regina. That's how we became friends. After your mother died and I sold my business and retired to Tampa Bay, Harv spent the winters with me. We were companions and L-O-V-E-R-S.

Remember the Christmas of 1980? The condo he had "rented"? It was <u>my</u> condo and I stayed in a goddamn hotel room. We had a fight of Titanic proportions over his refusal to tell you about <u>us</u>. We almost broke up. He was fearful you'd disown him. At the Christmas Eve service, I sat in the pew behind you, wished both of you a Merry Christmas and acted as if Harv were a perfect stranger.

I attended his funeral with my daughter Beth, sat with the collar of my topcoat pulled up, managed to hold in my sobs. I couldn't go to the interment, I would have lost it for sure. I said my goodbye in private at the

Green Groves Funeral Home the day before, and will visit his gravesite in my own time. Am I resentful? YES. Angry? YOU BET! Excuse my Bitch Karl voice (B-Boy. I-in. T-total. C-control. O-of. H-himself.), but a widower writes the obituary, leads the processional into the church, chooses the eulogist and pallbearers, receives flowers and sympathy cards honouring his long and devoted relationship and (DARE I MENTION?) an inheritance and survivor benefits?

When you cleaned out his apartment before going back to your ivory tower in Vancouver, you must've found *Xtra* magazines in his night table and God knows what else. Letters from me?

Monsieur Professeur, j'aimerais vous presenter . . . Harvey Sinclair Woods, your father. He made a mean Mexican omelette, gave the best back scratches, believed in God, called me KJ. We were good together. I am bereft.

Karl J. Werner

———

March 31, 1990
Stewart:
Got your letter.

There once was a doctor named Freud,
Who was probably mad, paranoid,
To him, always sex
Was a problem, a hex,
A thing to be cured, not enjoyed.

Harv felt he couldn't come out in Regina in the seventies, being a retired MLA. Plus he didn't want to embarrass you at the beginning of your academic career. What pisses me off is that he didn't tell you himself.

I came out thirty years ago when I left my wife. I told my son and daughter, "I'm a fag, like it or lump it. You live your lives, I'll live mine."

Are you in the same shoes, except yours are neatly lined up on the floor of your closet? Harv suspected you were gay when you continued to have *room-mates* long after you'd paid off your student loans and could afford a place of your own.

So your old man was gay . . . tough titty! Life is full of surprises and this one is not a delightful clown popping out of a jack-in-the-box.

This morning my old jack-in-the-box
Popped out and wouldn't get back-in-the-box

Karl

———

April 30, 1990

Stewart:

I'm just a soul whose intentions are good
Oh Lord, please don't let me be misunderstood

One phone call on your birthday and one phone call at Christmas does not constitute a relationship. The way I see it, the two of you were playing a game of Chicken. The principle of the game (in case you don't know) is that each player refuses to yield to the other, and as a result, the worst possible outcome occurs. In the case of you and Harv, the outcome was estrangement.

When he pitched the idea of the two of you paying your respects at your grandfather's grave on the 70th anniversary of The Battle of Vimy Ridge, you told him you couldn't possibly get away. Your grandfather was your namesake. You found time in your jam-packed schedule to gallivant around the globe on wine-tasting escapades, but you couldn't humour your old man by going to France with him. Incidentally, he intended to tell you about *us* on that trip.

During our last winter together, he came up with the idea of meeting you at the Montreal Jazz Festival. He said the one interest you shared was your love of jazz and blues. I don't know if he mustered the courage to mention it.

By the way, he told me about your illegitimate son. Uh-oh, another jack jumps out of the box! The boy must be in his thirties by now.

Mairzy doats and dozy doats
and little lambsy divey.
A kiddly ivey too,
wouldn't you?
Karl

———

May 18, 1990

Stewart:

Harv was proud of you. It is for you to decide if you can be proud of him.

He told me you encouraged your mother's love of horticulture and the piano, and were a devoted son during her final illness. He kept a copy of your book *Reappraising*

Colonialism in our living room and would show it to our guests. He said you had distanced yourself from your roots, that you were ashamed to say you were from Vagina, Saskatchewan.

Until the mid-seventies, Harv was more or less satisfied with his life — business, politics, family — that is until he came to terms with his repressed homosexuality.

It's hell on the prairies
such a shortage of fairies.

During his last winter here in Tampa Bay, he went to the racetrack most days and to church on Sundays. He played the stock market. He valued the fraternity of Masons.

Amor et melle et felle est fecundissimus. Love is rich with both honey and venom.

Karl

———

Four Fridays

#1

"WELL, LOOK WHAT THE CAT DRUG IN. How are ya?" Ruby is balancing two platters heaped with cheeseburgers and fries.

Richard's eyes are on the gapes in her blue uniform top. "Can't complain and if I did you wouldn't listen anyways." He straightens up the best he can and heads for his table in the corner. He throws his parka on the extra chair, sets himself down, takes off his John Deere cap, runs his fingers through what little hair he has left, puts his cap back on. Every Friday at 12:30, you can find him right here at the Husky Truck Stop, "original home of the pork chop sandwich". That's what it says on the sign out front.

"What can I get ya today, Dick?"

"The special."

"Which one? The breaded veal cutlets?"

"You musta read my mind."

"Be right back with coffee."

He's in town anyway, might as well put on the feedbag. At home, he eats straight out of the frying pan.

"Fill-er-up and don't forget . . . tomato juice insteada soup."

Richard used to be a regular on Thursdays, ate with Oskar Tollefson. Every blasted time, the Norwegian would bring up a meeting back in '57 in a place called Pugwash. Some scientists were talking about thermonuclear weapons threatening civilization (whatever thermonuclear means). The only meetings Richard ever went to were at the Lone Tree No. 18 R.M. office in Climax when he bitched about the grader leaving a big windrow across his driveway. Most times, when Tollefson got carried away with his Commie notions, all Richard would have to say was "Cat piss!" and change the subject, but that final Thursday when Tollefson wouldn't give Pugwash a rest, Richard up and left without dessert and switched his goin'-to-town-day to Fridays. The wife don't know the difference.

He's sizing up the couple in his line of vision. The man's skinny as a rake and the woman's a fatso. Even after Richard's seven-aught years on this earth, one thing he hasn't figured out is how people find each other. Him and Lyda went to the same one-room country schoolhouse, Anemone School. *An-em-on-ee*, but everyone pronounced it *An-enemy*. Look over yonder, Lardo is reaching for her husband's plate and wolfing down his leftover food. If she drops dead of a heart attack, Richard is willing to bet Jack Sprat will be looking for an easy keeper the second time around.

Not to say it was a match made in heaven for him and Lyda. He was the provider and she was the housekeeper. She cut out a picture of a chesterfield and chair in the catalogue, but he said their old furniture still had wear left in it. And she had the idea of painting the outside of the house yellow with white trim, called it "fixing the place up". He gave the barn and granaries a fresh coat of red that summer, told Lyda you don't take and put good money on the house. Machinery and farm buildings come first. At least that's how he sees things and it's him who controls the purse strings.

She threatened to leave him umpteen times, every year after the Farmers' Bonspiel Friday Night Smoker, guaranteed. Where would she have gone anyways? Couldn't go home to Mother because Mother was dead. Didn't have any money of her own to speak of, just the baby bonus. Richard used to tell her, "There's the door if you don't like it here. I can manage on my own." Funny thing, that's just what he's doing now, managing on his own with her in the Palliser.

"Here ya go."

"Looks fit for eatin'." Richard is a fan of good old meat and potatoes.

"How's Lyda?"

"About the same."

Lyda used to be a pretty good housekeeper and not a half-bad cook. Richard watches that couple mosey out. She must be two axe handles wide, reminds him of a sow. And her husband's a little puppy dog bringing up the rear. He must have to tie a board to his ass.

Odd couples, Richard can think of a few. Husbands with too much female hormones and vice-versa, like God got the recipe mixed up. Take the Smiths. He has little roses in his cheeks like he's wearing rouge. When you're talking to him, he leans in close to be sure he catches your every word. And her with a man's voice. You'd think they're two brothers. They even wear matching curling sweaters. Richard calls them "The Coughdrop Brothers".

"Refill?"

"If it's free, I'll take it. And could you spare a little more cow?"

"You betcha."

Then there's the Bartletts. Richard can tell she wears the pants. She's built like a brick shithouse, has a fuzzy mustache and lips that push out when she talks. Push out and pull back like an arsehole. And him with that snub of a nose, breathy fairy voice and little *lithp*. If he sees you in the waiting room at the doctor's office, he says he hopes you're feeling better real soon. You can tell he's genuinely sorry about your piles or that fiery rash in a moist dark place.

"And there's Ivan Updike."

"Pardon?"

"Oh, Jiminy Cricket, I musta been talkin' to myself."

"Did you leave room for dessert?"

"Yep, raisin pie alamode."

Ivan Updike pumps gas at The Loaf and Jug. He's all soft and pudgy, gurgles his s's. "Want your truck windowz wazshed?" He's a mouth breather, likely sucked his thumb as a kid. Wears a fake diamond earring, but can't be a fag 'cause he's got a wife. Richard seen the two of them in the Co-op grocery store, broad shoulders, bellies hanging over their blue jeans, her seams about to burst in the behind. From the back, they look like a pair of football players. He heard somewhere that Ivan writes romantic poems.

"Romantic," Richard scoffs.

"Pardon me?"

"Ah never mind. Thanks for the pie."

Hormones. Richard figures it all boils down to hormones, how much of each a person is born with. But how do these odd people find each other? That's what he'd like to know. In his day, they would've been old maids or bachelors. Now they hook up, a tomboy and a pansy for instance. How does it work after they take off their pants and climb into bed for Chrissake? He'd like to know that, too.

Richard leaves a loonie beside his pie plate for Ruby. She's on her feet all day.

Outside, Nigger is barking his head off in the box of the half-ton. Before Richard climbs in, he blows his nose with his thumb. The snot lands in a snowbank.

#2

Richard shambles over to his table in the corner.

"How's life in the fast lane?" Ruby asks.

"Can't complain."

"What'll ya have?"

"The roast turkey."

"I'll be right back with coffee and your tomato juice."

"Thanks Ruby."

Richard's mechanically inclined, so he started up a little vehicle repair business, a sideline to cattle farming. The wife was still at home then. She nagged about his "junkyard". (That's what she called the used cars and machinery he keeps for parts.) Said she was sick and tired of looking out the kitchen window at his junkyard.

"Junkyard." He spits out the word.

"What's that?" Ruby asks.

"Must've been thinkin' out loud. Looks good."

"You'll like the stuffing. It's to die for."

The business was Richard's way of bringing in a little extra cash. There's always somebody running into car trouble on the

Number 1, so he put up a sign on the quarter-section along the highway: "Dick's Service, Climax, Phone 293-6728". A few travellers did stop, paid him cash for his trouble. Three or four neighbours brought their grain trucks for tune-ups. It was good, except the sign made him a laughing stock around Climax. He should've seen it coming, but he didn't.

"Plum pudding? Comes with the turkey dinner."

"You bet."

He thought about changing the sign to "Richard's Service" or "Dick's Vehicle Repairs", but be damned if he was gonna give them boozers at The Bijou any satisfaction. He calls them "old women", the way they gossip.

"Yeah, I'll have one more refill."

One of them sneaky bastards took a picture of his sign and sent it to *The Leader Post*, and would you believe they published it? He doesn't get the paper, but the clipping came in the mail in an envelope with no return address. He took his sign down in harvest when nobody would be paying any attention, then started doing his shopping in Swift Current instead of Climax. It means an extra 120 miles of driving, which is why he goes only once a week. With the wife in the Palliser, he can kill two birds with one stone.

"How's Lyda?" Ruby asks.

"About the same."

"I was at the Palliser singing with my church. Kinda breaks your heart, all those elderly people in their wheelchairs. Some of 'em can't even lift their heads."

"Don't hardly notice anymore."

"I just hope and pray it won't be me someday. I told my old man, 'Take me out behind the barn and shoot me if I lose my marbles.'" Ruby picks the drumstick bone off the table and puts it on Richard's plate, gathers up his water glass and cutlery. "Sorry, I guess I put my foot in my mouth."

"Don't matter."

They take good care of Richard's wife at the Palliser. She's always clean and the girls seem kind-hearted. It's been seven years since she went outside in the middle of the night without a winter coat or boots. Richard followed her to the machine shed, grabbed her to make her turn around, but she was bound and determined she was going to her sister Dolly's for a baby shower. He had to get rough with her before she'd come back into the house, left a bruise on her arm. "The final straw", that's what their daughter said. It was time for Mother to go into a home.

Driving back to the farm, Richard thinks maybe he should've done what Ruby said, took Lyda out behind the barn and shot her. It might've been more humane than letting her linger. A farmer has to have the nerve to shoot a dog that bites or a suffering cow. He can't be phoning the vet every time to put the animal down.

#3

Richard didn't bother to change out of his barn clothes this morning after he did chores. There's manure stuck to his gum boots.

"Guess you can tell I'm not retired yet," he says to Ruby.

"Retired, tired, or retarded?"

"A little of each."

They both laugh.

"What'll ya have?" Ruby asks.

"Maybe I'll have the pork chop sandwich t'day."

"With fries?"

"Why not? Gravy on the side."

Ruby's got a nice ass. Richard wishes he could see it bare. Puts him in mind of that winter him and Lyda went south. One afternoon, he took *The Western Producer* and a glass of Pepsi, slid open the patio doors of their suite and stepped outside. Their balcony was paired up with the suite next door, two balconies side by side looking out over a swimming pool. A woman was suntanning in a two-piece bathing suit on one of those lounge chairs no more than six feet away. She must've been fifty years old, but still had a terrific pair of tits. They both said hello and Richard told her his wife went to a quilt show with some ladies from back home and she said her husband was a golfing fanatic and she was bored to tears. She fake-yawned, patting her open mouth with the palm of her hand and spelled out B-O-R-E-D. He blocked the view with his newspaper and pretended to read. After a while, he went inside to refill his glass, and when he came out, she was lying on her stomach buck naked. There were beads of sweat all over her greasy body. He could feel movement in his boxer shorts. Next thing, she scrunched up on the lounge chair so that her ass was in the air facing him. He'd seen female dogs in heat doing that, turning their backside toward a male and inviting him to mount. It's called presenting.

He must've spoken out loud because Ruby asked, "Did you say presenting?"

"Nah."

"Brought you some extra applesauce. How's Lyda?"

"About the same."

He waited for his hard-on to fade that sunny afternoon, then went inside. There was a little dribble in his underwear, so he changed and sat down in front of the television. That woman was asking for it, no question. These days, the only attention his dink gets is when Nigger noses under the blankets and gives it a lick on his way to the foot of the bed. The picture is still clear in his mind, her round pink bum with that little tuft of hair peeking through the crack.

He pays for his meal, makes a stop at the Co-op, then Peavey Mart, and hits the road, thinking the whole time about how there are some real strange people south of the border.

#4

It's 12:30 and Richards' heading for his table in the corner, regular as clockwork.

"How goes it, Dick?"

"Can't complain." He's gotta act like nothing's out of the ordinary.

"What'll ya have?"

"How 'bout the hamburger steak?"

"Okey-dokey. Be right back with the coffee."

The dining room at the Palliser will be emptying out about now. On Fridays, one of the girls always brings a tray to Lyda's room. Most of the food was still left on her plate when he gave up on trying to feed her. That's why she's down to eighty pounds. The teaspoon rattles against his mug. A little coffee slops over the edge when he lifts it up to his mouth.

He was telling Lyda about spraying Round-up along the road allowance. He scooped up some mashed potatoes, gravy, and a few crumbs of roast chicken, and touched the spoon to her lips till they quivered. When she opened her mouth a smidgeon, he put in the tip of the spoon and had to wait for her to open wider before he could nuzzle the spoon in the rest of the way. She coughed, so he pulled the spoon back out, but the food stayed in her mouth. She swallowed, then she gagged. He thought she was going to puke.

"Enjoy your meal," Ruby says.

"Will do." The truth is he doesn't have much of an appetite.

One minute Lyda gagged. The next minute she stopped breathing. He should've slapped her on the back or poked his finger down her throat, but he did absolutely nothing. He could've pushed the call button or hollered for help but he just sat there paralyzed, watching her face turn grey, then bluish. It didn't take long. She never struggled at all. She was too weak. After her head slumped onto her chest and she quit breathing, he slipped out of her room and exited the building. Drove across town to the Husky Truck Stop. It wasn't until he sat down at the table that he started to shake.

He puts a French fry in his mouth and gums it. It tastes like grease and salt. They would've found Lyda by now. Either a kitchen helper collecting the tray or an aide coming to change her diaper and put her to bed for an afternoon nap. A nurse would have to write something on a form. "Found dead in her wheel-chair at 12:30 PM Friday March 2, 2012." They're probably trying to reach him on the phone. He'll have to act surprised and upset. As a matter of fact, he is both surprised and upset. Granted, it had gone through his head plenty of times how he wished she was out of her misery, but he didn't plan it. It wasn't what they call pre-meditated. He swallows one French fry, then another.

"How about a refill, Dick?"

"No thanks." He pushes the food around on his plate.

"You've hardly touched your food. How's Lyda?"

He keeps his eyes on his plate. "About the same." He's shaking bad. He sets down the fork.

"You want me to box that up so you can take it home for supper?"

"Sure."

Ruby brings the box and some steak bones wrapped in a paper napkin for Nigger.

Showdown in Fort Benton

I'M TREATING MY WIFE TO A weekend in Fort Benton and it's not even her birthday or our anniversary. She was very impressed with the room I booked. It's their most expensive room. And I mean *high end*. It even has a balcony where they say ladies used to watch gunfights on Front Street. Plus we've got a view of two teepees pitched across the Upper Missouri River. After we checked in on Friday night, my wife soaked in the clawfoot tub and I toasted myself for coming up with such a brilliant idea.

Last night, we ate at The Union Grille. That's the name of the posh restaurant in our hotel. We had duck with a rice mixture and a pistachio sauce. Pricey, not a lot of food, but Sheila raved about it. The only time I ever tasted pistachio before, it was ice-cream in Waskesiu.

Sheila said not to splurge again tonight, so we're at Bob's Riverfront Café. It's the only eating establishment that isn't a pub. The Sunday special is hamburger steak, beverage and dessert included, for $11.99. Some country and western crooner is going on and on about how he's gonna pay the rent.

Yesterday, when we walked by, there were people at every table, but tonight we're the only customers. There's football on

TV, so folks must've eaten early and hurried home. I wish I could watch the game myself. Chicago at Atlanta.

A man in a wrinkled white shirt and dirty apron is slumped over the bar, sipping on a coffee.

Sheila leans across the table and lowers her voice. "Do you think that's Bob?"

"Must be."

Bob tells the waitress and the boy-chef he's going home, and disappears into the back.

It's not hard to see and do everything there is to see and do in Fort Benton in one weekend. This morning, my wife wanted to walk on this path along the riverbank that goes from one end of town to the other, so I agreed. She insisted on stopping to read every damn sign. As for myself, I was partial to the statues, larger-than-life, of whiskey traders and Indians, businessmen and scoundrels. We sat for a while on these benches they put on the old railroad bridge, watched some whooping cranes land and take off.

We should've been served by now, but the solo waitress is on the phone checking up on her kids.

Next to our table there's an antique buffet with a fancy silver coal-oil lamp. Glass bits dangle from the shade like a chandelier. Sheila gets up to take a closer look at the picture of Nez Perce Chief Joseph. She says, "It was *his* rifle we saw on display."

"Yeah, confiscated by the US Cavalry."

Yesterday, at the Interpretive Centre, we learned all about the Battle of Bear Paw. We also found out there are paddlefish dating back to the dinosaur age, in the Missouri River They're the ugliest fish you've ever seen. When we were inside the steamboat pilot house, my wife whispered, "I think that's enough education for me for one day." A knowing wink wink signalled her interest in a lie-down on our king-sized bed at the hotel. I was feeling a little frisky myself.

Sheila asks, "Have you eaten here before?"

I'm getting aroused thinking about us having sex yesterday afternoon plus both nights, and how it's looking good for tonight. "No, I never ate anywhere. I just stayed at that hotel that looks like a furniture store."

"Yeah, you showed me."

The place was a rabbit warren. In the morning, an old lady in a kimono, with her hair in curlers, said, "Mornin. Coffee's made. The Lord helps them that helps themselves." Her and these two old men were sitting close enough to a little filing cabinet to reach the thermos of coffee, a can of milk, and sugar cubes. One of them, who looked like he'd just climbed out of bed, asked, "Where ya from?" It was a scene from an Alfred Hitchcock movie. Their definition of a continental breakfast consisted of a package of sticky buns with white icing, a few missing. I went back to my room, poured the styrofoam cup of coffee down my sink, grabbed my suitcase, gave the trio a "so-long" and left.

I say to my wife, "This café is halfway between the only two hotels. Our dinner last night and the breakfast pastries at the far end of the street must be the extremes."

We're laughing about that when the waitress hollers at us from behind the bar. "Menus?" She's off the phone.

"Yes please," I holler back.

"Two waters?"

"Yeah."

"With ice?"

"Sure." Then I say to Sheila, "Back in April, when I set foot in the Grand Union, I felt like I'd walked into a bygone era."

"It's a jewel hidden in backwoods Montana. *Cowboy Victorian*, that's what they call the decor. The only thing missing is a mature hostess in a skin-tight red gown . . . " Sheila uses both hands to outline a curved figure from top to bottom. " . . . elbow-length black gloves, her hair in a French roll, and a beauty mark on her cheek, beckoning guests into the bar."

I chuckle.

"Oh, and a guy with lambchop sideburns, a three-piece suit, and a pocket watch, reading a newspaper on that leather couch in the lobby."

The Grand Union should hire my wife to write their brochures. She's hinted at making this an annual romantic getaway. After twenty-eight years, things are a little stale, so I'm all for it.

"I knew you'd like this town." I say.

"Especially the way they've preserved their history, albeit violent."

"There mustn't be any zoning bylaws — bungalows next door to shanties, and trailers stuck in here and there."

The waitress is high-spirited, about the same age as Melissa, in jeans and a T-shirt, short hair sticking up. I glance at her name tag, "Lisa", but avoid the slogan across her chest.

"Where ya from?" Lisa asks. Quite a contrast from our classy waitress last night. I can't help noticing her figure. She tells us she works two jobs, the other at a gas station, and never sees her kids on weekends. I'm not sure if she's bragging, complaining, or vying for a tip. The soundtrack to her hardluck story is booming through the speaker, something about a wife dreamin' of a house on the hill.

Sheila orders a glass of red wine and I order a beer.

Five minutes later, Lisa delivers our plates with mounds of food. "Eat up."

We haven't had time to finish our drinks.

"What time do you close?" I ask.

"Soon, but don't rush. We've gotta do the clean-up."

"I'll have another beer."

I've taken a few bites of my hamburger steak when the door swings open and in swaggers a black cowboy hat, a black muscle shirt and tight black jeans, bulging biceps, tattoos from shoulder to wrist, and a hunting knife tucked into a belt sheath in the middle of her back. She saunters over to a barstool, mounts it like it was a horse, and says to Lisa, "Coors and a rib-eye like usual." She spins her stool ninety degrees and raises one cowboy boot up onto the next stool. Legs apart, one knee bent. A flirt with a little dirt. The same CD is playing, must be on repeat.

Lisa's demeanour changes. There's a cock to her head and a wiggle to her bum. She sets down a tall glass in front of the customer and pours in a bottle of beer, then disappears into the kitchen. We can hear her say to the boy-chef, "Shove over. I know how she likes her steaks." Through a wicket window, Lisa and the cowgirl banter back and forth while the grill sizzles. Suddenly Lisa lets out a squeal, then laughs loudly and explains that the chef got her wet, " . . . but not in a good way."

The lean mean chick slides down from her stool, slips behind the bar, helps herself to a take-out cup, and dumps in her beer. She barks at Lisa, "I'm not takin' any more of your bullshit," and heads for the door. She jerks it open, sucking in a gust of cold air. We can see her through the window, climbing into a black Dodge Ram 1500 and taking a gulp of beer.

Lisa walks right past us and takes a wide-legged stance facing the window straight on. Are we about to witness a showdown at dusk? According to the tourist brochures, Front Street used to be the bloodiest block in the West.

Hands on hips, Lisa blurts out, "Well . . . are ya gonna pull them pistols or are ya justa whistlin' Dixie?" as if she could be heard from outside. I wait for rodeo gal to dismount from her black Ram and whoop Lisa's ass, but instead she backs up out of her parking stall, then lays a strip of rubber. She passes the statue of the faithful collie Shep, then the Grand Union Hotel, then heads east toward Geraldine. My wife and I follow her tail lights across the bridge over the National Wild and Scenic Upper Missouri River.

Modern Apparel

Luck

MIRIAM WAITS UNTIL THE OTHER PASSENGERS exit the bus. Then she uses the pole to pull herself to a standing position, grips the handrail, and watches her shoes step down to the sidewalk. She can't afford to slip and fall. At the bus stop, men shift their weight from one foot to the other. They're skinny, grizzled smokers with necks wrapped in scarves and briefcases poking out of their armpits. The girls in leggings look to Miriam like they've forgotten their skirts at home. She walks along *Avenue Bernard* in Outrement, with people rushing past her on both sides.

She stops at Modern Apparel, rises onto her tippy-toes, pulls envelopes and flyers out of the mailbox, and unlocks the door. The paper with the words *Logement A Louer* is still where she pasted it to the window of the separate entrance accessing the second storey.

Fluorescent tubes running the length of the store light up. Some of them flicker. Miriam throws her coat over a rack, and makes her way past the merchandise to a congested little office.

Today only, she unlocks the back door. Then, as if performing an Orthodox ritual, she fiddles with the bent key to unlock the filing cabinet, then removes the cash drawer, then carries it to the front of the store and slides it into the cash register. The same pattern for opening the store every day, the same steps done precisely the same way.

Then she sits down behind the counter and dials the telephone. "Hello." She inhales through her nose and opens her chest as if she's preparing for yoga, then exhales before speaking the next words. "This is Miriam Lis. I am getting *The Gazette*."

"You know pensioners can't anymore afford it, the price went up so much."

"So what is the best price you can give for me?"

"I want it from Monday to Saturday. It doesn't come anyways on Sunday."

"Well if you can't do me something, I have to cancel it." She hangs up.

In keeping with her store-opening ritual, she goes over to a chrome chair facing the picture window and lowers herself onto the vinyl seat with stuffing poking out. Behind her, yellowed cardboard boxes are stacked, each one the size of two pounds of butter. It is 12:00 noon and Modern Apparel is open for business.

Montrealers bustle past, oblivious to Miriam observing them, or nodding off on her watch. Today, the bell rings and the first customer comes through the door earlier than usual, before Miriam even has time to get settled into her chair. It's a young woman wearing a black leather jacket, carcoat length, with a colourful scarf, mostly purple, wrapped around her neck twice, then tucked into the collar. There's nothing special about her except for her purse. It's purple, too, with silver-coloured chains for handles.

Miriam edges forward and asks the woman, "How can I help you?"

The blonde-haired woman squints to adjust to the dim light, locates Miriam, and says, "I'm looking for panties." She acts as if she has no time to waste.

Miriam gets up with some effort and leads the way down the aisle past a rack of pastel dresses to a cramped corner with odds and ends of lingerie — white flannelette pyjamas with blue snowflakes, a wine-coloured velour bathrobe, and a bin of brassieres and panties. Two men from a maintenance company come in through the back door while the customer is rifling through the underwear — dented boxes with white 24-hour Playtex brassieres guaranteed not to pinch or slip, packages of sensible panties. Junior is carrying a ladder, Senior a fluorescent tube. Miriam tells them the building is an old beast continually demanding repairs. She points upstairs and says "dripping, dripping, dripping" three times, the tenant says it's driving him nuts, he threatens to move out, bad enough there's one empty apartment, never mind both.

After the ladder is set up, Junior grabs the bulb from Senior. The customer, package in hand, takes a detour around the ladder, proceeds to the front counter, and waits. Miriam offers some appreciation to Junior, who is using both arms to press a four foot long bulb into a ceiling fixture. Senior presumably has disappeared upstairs to investigate the drip.

The customer tries to start a conversation, but Miriam is distracted, her eyes flitting from Junior up the ladder, to the back entrance, anxious for Senior to reappear. The customer pays for her panties, pans the store, and leaves.

The next day, she comes back and introduces herself as Alanna Hildermann from Regina, Saskatchewan, and explains that she's in Montreal for a nurses' meeting. She asks Miriam, "I was wondering which part of Europe you immigrated from."

Miriam bristles as if Alanna just slapped her, as if this happens every day, people coming into her store, buttering her up, asking a bunch of nosy questions, bothering her. She puts an abrupt end to it. "I am a Holocaust survivor and I do not want to talk about it."

"Oh dear, I had no idea." Alanna's presumptuousness dissolves, her mouth widens, and her neck tightens into a contorted expression of horror. "Honest, it's you I'm interested in, you and this store."

"I don't want to be public. Many opportunities I have to tell my story." Miriam has put Alanna in her place. Subject closed.

"Yes of course. I understand."

But does Alanna understand? Besides the Holocaust, what else is there about Miriam and Modern Apparel that could possibly be of interest? That she grew up in the Carpathian Mountains of Romania, which was later annexed by Hungary? That her father owned a mill called Giller Textiles, in the village of Sighet? That the war interrupted Miriam's first year of university?

The people in Sighet were civil to each other, but a man who lived across the street from Gillers let it slip, unknowingly forewarning them. "We want all the other Jews taken away except for your family." That's what he said to Miriam. *Taken away.* But Gillers did not heed the warning. There came an insistent knock on their door and they were herded into a ghetto on Serpent Street, along with all of the other Jews in their town. Three months later, soldiers loaded them onto a train to Auschwitz-Birkenau.

"*Aufstehen! Aufstehen! Wstac!*" It's been sixty-seven years, but when Miriam first awakens in the morning, she can hear the matron shouting in the Lager, her lips barely parted, giving commands. She was a brute, that one, her dishwater blonde hair waved and slicked back, her erect spine, thick ankles, chin raised. Miriam would sit up, her heart would race, she would grab her shoes if they hadn't been stolen, look over to be sure Bronia was up, make the *bettenbau* with hospital corners over a shapeless straw mattress, and run outside for the basin shared by hundreds. Cold water was better than none. She would line up for roll call, checking for Bronia again. It was 4:00 AM.

The matron would beat stragglers, knock them to the ground. If a captive looked at her *the wrong way*, she'd single her out, never to be seen again. She'd cull the sickly ones who couldn't work, and send them to the gas chambers without even blinking. She was evil, and evil isn't always wearing pants. Was she saving her own skin? To the contrary, Miriam could tell she relished her power. What did the matron get out of it? The privilege of sleeping with one of the officers? Being his *prietenă*.

On the rare occasion when Miriam talked about Auschwitz, all she said was, "I was a slave in the Union Factory." No details were offered. She left it to the listener to imagine the IG Farben-Bayer chemical factory, *IG Farbenindustrie*. The work was hard and often useless, moving heavy containers from Point A to Point B, doing everything fast, no slowing down, with insults and beatings from the *kapos*, afternoons tougher than mornings because of hunger, and on the march back to the Lagers, maybe the guards would order the slaves to sing.

Lining up, always lining up, for roll-call, for bread, to go to the factories. But one morning was different. The women were ordered to take their bowl and spoon, and follow the male prisoners on a march to another camp, stopping at a barn along the way to sleep on a stone floor covered with straw, like pigs. In the morning, lining up again and marching to the next camp and the next, stepping over prisoners who fell and would be left to freeze to death. Miriam tried, but couldn't look away, when a guard shot the woman ahead of her and kicked her body into a ditch. On another day of marching, she was ordered to carry a dead body to the next camp for evening roll-call. The only hope came when she saw Yaron. At least one of her brothers was still alive. After the war, she learned the reason for this parade of stick people, the Death March. The Nazis knew the Red Army was crowding in.

When the ruthless matron and the other guards fled, Miriam, Bronia, and Yaron huddled together. They were free to go, but where? And how? Then the American soldiers arrived, sent from Heaven, and transported the prisoners to a DP camp.

Wouldn't the prying customer like to know all of this? Including the juiciest tidbit of all, that Miriam's parents, another sister, and another brother perished in the gas chambers.

Miriam met Sydney Lis in the DP camp. After they married, they lived in Sweden. That was where Miriam read in a newspaper

that the matron from Auschwitz was hanged at the age of twenty-
six for war crimes.

Miriam and Sydney moved from Sweden to Israel, then
put down roots in Montreal, working in the garment and rag
industry along with other Romanian people. Bronia made her
home in Israel, Yaron in Sweden. None of them ever returned to
Romania. The Gillers were the Diaspora.

Since Sydney's heart attack eleven years ago, Miriam has
been walking across a skating rink in slippery-soled shoes with
no boards to hang onto. So far she has managed to stay upright.
Yes, she has the business and her children, grandchildren, even
her first great-grandchild, but they can't take the place of her
sweetheart Sydney, her go-to-sleep-with-me, wake-up-beside-
me, grow-old-with-me Sydney.

The nurse from Regina is back after a year. Or is it longer?
She reminds Miriam of her name, even spells it for her. A-L-A-
N-N-A. She buys a pair of slacks and has the nerve to ask, "Do
you ever think about retiring?"

"What would I all the time do at home? I have no housework.
A woman cleans my house every Thursday. An immigrant
from Romania. I go home to fresh ironed sheets and the faucets
polished. My son says to me, 'How long you are going to be
janitor?' He thinks I should sell off this building."

"You're not a janitor," Alanna interjects. "You're a landlady."

Miriam is testy. "No, I am *not* a landlady. I don't want to be
sooperior."

"I mean, you rent out apartments."

"I am a business person. $8000 it cost for me to upgrade one of the apartments last year." She raises her eyebrows and her shoulders as if to say, "*C'est la vie.*" It's all part of doing business.

"I noticed all the buttons you have," Alanna says. "Your wall of buttons. You must be in love with buttons."

Miriam covers her mouth and laughs at such a ridiculous comment. "No, I don't think so I'm in love with buttons."

Then Alanna starts talking about Elie Wiesel, of all people. Miriam's famous cousin. His sister Hilda was in the same Lager with her and Bronia. To curtail the conversation and hurry Alanna on her way, Miriam gathers her purse and coat, and says, "It's Friday."

She will close early for Shabbat, which begins at sunset and will end at sunset tomorrow when three stars appear in the sky. Miriam loves her Shabbat. She does not work, cook, or travel. That's the law for Orthodox Jews. To her, these laws are like mountains hanging by a hair. She will stay home, light candles, and read, but she will not go to a synagogue to pray. How could she be expected to believe that God answers prayers?

"Do you still have nightmares?" Alanna asks.

A brazen question, but Miriam answers it. "No, it's blacked out. I have a strong character. It's luck. Some of us were lucky to get out. Some were not."

Alanna buttons up her coat, slings her purse over her shoulder, and walks out onto *Avenue Bernard*. Miriam's survival had nothing whatsoever to do with luck and everything to do with grace.

When Miriam gets home, she discovers her wallet is missing from her purse. People coming and going from the store, teenagers wanting fabric for their Home economics projects, it could have been any one of them. The next day, the wallet reappears in the mailbox at the store. He must have been a kind-hearted thief, she thinks. Either that or he got cold feet. No money is missing, but the idea that a stranger went through her purse and knows her address, gives her a bad feeling. It's no use phoning the police. The last time she talked to them, it was about a drug dealer who owned the store across the street and kept a gun on the counter. The officer wanted to use Miriam's upstairs suite to spy on him, but she refused, saying she didn't need trouble. The drug dealer has since died, his store is boarded up, and his heirs or creditors are fighting over the property.

A letter comes from Jerusalem, from Bronia's daughter, Ruth. Not even a letter, just a note. "We had to put Mother in *Ahuzat Beit HaKerem* Rehabilitation Home. She fell. Only bruises, no broken bones. She says if you want to see her alive you better come. *Shalom*, Ruth."

Bronia has never understood why Miriam won't join her in the Promised Land. She has early dementia and keeps repeating the same questions in Yiddish. "Where's Miriam?" "Where's Montreal?" "They speak French there, don't they?" Miriam has no intention of leaving Montreal. Her first two children were born in Sweden, the third in Canada, and now that she is widowed with all of her children living close-by, the die has been cast. *Zol zein.* Of course, she wishes she had a closer relationship with Bronia and Yaron, but like most brothers and sisters, they've bickered, and the few times they've dared to talk about their childhood and the war, each of them remembers things differently.

Miriam's grandson, long-haired Simon Rosen, studies Chemistry at McGill. He volunteered for the summer on an Israeli kibbutz. Fired up by Zionism and *Yad Vashem*, he had Miriam's concentration camp ID number tattooed on his wrist. *A12989*. He sought out his Israeli relatives. Great-Aunt Bronia swooned when he exposed his tattoo. After all, she is a frail, quavering resident in a care home. In faltering Yiddish, he tried to explain his intention to honour his grandmother's suffering in Auschwitz. Just as he raised his arm to block Bronia from falling forward out of her wheelchair, her daughter Ruth arrived. Bronia's head was hanging in her lap. She was moaning.

"What is going on here?" Ruth pushed Simon aside. "You come from Canada all the way here to upset an old lady?"

Simon's pilgrimage ended on a sour note. He returned to Montreal with more questions about his heritage than answers. His mother, Luba, explained why Bronia was so upset. After Auschwitz, Bronia gave birth to a daughter out of wedlock and named her Luba. Miriam, who was married with one child already, agreed to raise Luba as her own. Bronia, not Miriam, is Simon's biological grandmother and her ID number is *A12990*. Simon had been tattooed with the wrong number. All Miriam could do when this news reached her was shrug her shoulders and throw up her hands. "*Oi, Vay!* Such a pity! A young man what got so disappointed, the grandmothers mixed together for him."

Some things, like Simon's tattoo, Miriam doesn't understand. But some things she knows. Harper's government, spending all the time spending, millions on airplanes and children go hungry, he treats Jews nice as long as they vote for him, he shouldn't treat one group special, Indians — what about the Indians with not a proper house? It's the law in the Torah how to make harmony. In the Bible too, not? Better he should be feeding hungry children. This is *The Manifesto of Miriam Lis*.

It is Friday evening and Miriam is soaking in bathwater with almond oil. Her thoughts drift from Shabbat to her Sydney to her mother. She can't remember her mother's voice. She knows that her mother called her "M" only because Yaron reminded her.

After towel-drying, she dabs underneath each breast and between her legs with a Rose-scented powder puff. She pulls on a thin nylon nightgown, brushes her hair back, cleanses her face with cold cream, applies moisturizer, and brushes her teeth. She coaxes her hammer toes into worn slippers and pads down the hallway to her bedroom, passing gas.

To Miriam, the house (with the exception of her bedroom) is a void. She pulls the string on the lamp on her night table, drapes the bedspread over a chair, folds back the blanket and top sheet, sits on the bed, and takes off her slippers. Her reading glasses are beside *Prague Winter*. Most evenings, she reads until she's drowsy, but how can she read tonight with her mother on her mind? Usually, she replays in the dark her conversations with Sydney. Their fifty-five year dialogue she can remember, but how it feels to make love, she can't. Tonight, she turns off the lamp and snuggles into her cozy nest. On her left side with her knees pulled up, one hand under the pillow and the other in a fist under her chin, she closes her eyes and concentrates on her mother. How many times, how many hundreds of times has she tried to visualize her? What could be more pitiable than forgetting your own mother's face? It was the customer's remark about buttons, a joke really, that coaxed a memory to Miriam's consciousness. She can see her mother's cape. Not her face, only her cape. The cape she was wearing the last time Miriam saw her step down from the train. A pink cashmere cape fastened with one fuchsia button. Miriam can see the button, the splendid beauty of it.

Buttons

Noise, crazy drivers, litter. That was my first impression of Montreal. Pizza boxes, mattresses, splintered lumber, even toilets for Christ's sake had been left at the curb. In Outrement, not only the Hasidic Jews, but everyone was wearing black.

I went to Montreal for a nurses' clinical conference. That was four years ago. I represented the Regina Qu'appelle Health Region. It was early November and the tires of my taxi cab crunched through autumn leaves piled high on a narrow street on the way to *L'Auberge Bouchard*. Madame Bouchard showed me to my room, cluttered with Victorian *frou frou*. After I freshened up, she pointed me in the direction of a store because Air Canada lost my suitcase.

"Modern Apparel" was etched on the window. When I opened the door, a bell clanged and I heard, "How can I help you?" The croaky little voice belonged to an old woman sitting off to one side facing the window. People-watching I guess.

"I'm looking for panties," I said, and that's how it all began, my connection to Miriam Lis, the elderly owner of this elderly store. Over time, things spun out of control.

Although the store was called *Modern* Apparel, its merchandise was from the turn of the century, not the last turn, but the turn before. Stale air. Deadly silence. Zero ambiance. I couldn't figure out why M. Bouchard would recommend such a crap store.

I rummaged through a wire mesh bin of panties in crumpled packages and bras in dented boxes, and pulled out a three-pack of Granny gitch. Pink, white, and blue cotton. Pre-Spandex, maybe even pre-nylon. I hadn't worn cotton undies since public school, but what choice did I have? I'd had to go commando because my only pair was drying on a towel rack at the B & B, and there weren't any other clothing stores in sight.

Somewhere in my memory bank there's a shopping trip with my mother to a cluttered department store that smelled musty. The main floor was jam-packed with clothing and shoes for women, men, and children, and in the basement there were pillows, bedding, towels, and knick knacks.

Mum tried on dresses, pulling back the curtain of the change stall to model each one timidly in front of a three-way mirror. The salesclerk's grey hair was pulled back into a bun. It wasn't rinsed with Soft Brown capsules and permed like Mum's. I watched her cherry red lips *ooh* and *aah* while she adjusted the shoulder pads or tucked the waist to demonstrate how alterations could improve the fit. Meanwhile I was squirming on a velvet-covered bench, taking it all in. When Mum finally exited the change stall with her coat buttoned up and only her purse in hand, the clerk put on pressure. "But Mrs. Hildermann, this one was made for you." (Somehow she knew my mother's name.) "It's perfect," she said, and thrust one of the dresses, a black crepe with a metallic gold cumberbund, which I thought was glamourous, toward Mum. "Take it home on approval why don't you?" She smacked her red mouth as if she was savouring something sweet and sticky. "At least see what your husband says," she coaxed, but my mother said meekly, "I'd like to think it over." I felt a let's-get-out-of-here-right-this-minute nudge in the small of my back. There was perspiration on Mum's forehead.

Dad was waiting outside in the car because Mum didn't drive. "No parcels?" he said.

"Never mind let's go home," she huffed. "That's the last time I go into that Jew store."

"Cash only," the proprietor of Modern Apparel said, in spite of a cluster of stickers — Visa, MasterCard, Interac, American Express — on the antiquated cash register. She lifted her glasses hanging from a gold chain on her bosom, and put them on. Her eyebrows were beansprouts.

"This must be your store, is it?"

She was concentrating on the transaction. "I am the manager."

"Oh."

She leaned toward the cash register, then moved her face even closer, to focus on pushing the right buttons. The liver spots on her cheeks were the size of nickels.

"I'm Alanna Hildermann."

ChChing.

"From Regina, Saskatchewan."

No response.

"May I ask your name?"

"Miriam."

"When did you start working here?

"I don't remember."

I was dying to find out where she came from and how long she'd been in that outdated store, but she got all prickly when I asked any questions. Her fingers, zigzagged with osteoarthritis, struggled to put my purchase into a plastic bag. I considered offering to do it for her, but didn't want to make her feel self-conscious. Instead I struck up a conversation about whether it was likely to rain or not.

She said, "Vee vill haff to vait and see." Her accent reminded me of my grandmother on my mother's side.

I was excited about my first out-of-province conference. All expenses paid. Over the course of three days, Montreal wormed its way into my heart. The walk-ups, the coffee shops, the *boulangeries*, the second-hand *fripperies*, the smoked meat delis, hearing French at every turn, but mostly I was smitten by Miriam, the stooped Jewess in her dingy shop.

I've heard a lot of life stories, enough to write a book, fill a bookshelf, even a phone booth if I put them all together. No two are the same, each has its ups and downs, the sad and the glad. Never the whole story. Censored. Embellished. Maybe not even the truth, the whole truth, and nothing but the truth so help me God. Some are even naughty. I used to write up the life stories of elders in the nursing home where I worked. It wasn't really part of my job, but old folks appreciate when someone takes the time to listen. I'd jot down a few facts — birthplace, marriage, children, etc, much like an obituary. Then I'd sprinkle in amusing anecdotes, like the time the farmer's wife mistook a pail of axle grease for jam, or the hired man who got fired after kicking over the traces the night before. I used the residents' own words as much as I could. If there was anything unpleasant or tragic, I'd make a brief reference to it, like the man who put his brother's name on a raffle ticket and, after his brother drove off with the car he won, the two never spoke to each other again. "Lars and his twin brother Linton are estranged." Or the woman who ran over her little boy when he fell out of their old jalopy and she drove over him. "Alex died in a car accident when he was only four years old." I left out some stuff, like the bosomy housewife who literally got her tits caught in the wringer, and the so-called mental defective whose mantra was, "Bastard bugger bitch baloney bastard bugger bitch baloney bastard bugger . . . " taught to him by his uncle. I printed the stories onto a sheet of paper with a fancy border and slipped them into a plastic page-protector. I'd make extra copies if residents asked.

I dropped in on Miriam two more times and she did tell me a few things. She was eighty-four and had managed the clothing store and two upstairs apartments for forty years. (I still don't understand why she calls herself the manager when she owns the building.) She is a widow, and whenever she says the name of her deceased husband Sydney, she squeezes her eyes shut. She has three children, six grandchildren, and one great-grandchild, but the only two she named are surgeons — Dr. David Rosen, her son-in-law, an internist, and Dr. Lenora Lis, her granddaughter, an oncologist.

I had to answer a few of her questions, too. Where was I from? Regina. Was I married? Yes, for ten years. Did I have children? No, Curtis and I chose not to have children. When I said that, Miriam raised her hands open-palmed. Baffled? Or was it pity? I'm not sure.

I made two more trips to Montreal. They're all blurred together — the chair with the ripped green vinyl upholstery, the buttons, the wallet, the Lager, her cousins. To pay for one of the trips, I withdrew money earmarked for a house payment. Curtis didn't find out until after I lost my job.

One cold drizzly November morning, I skulked around Modern Apparel before it opened. The long yellow plastic panels hanging in the show window are like the lenses in those cardboard 3D glasses we wore to watch Andy Warhol's *Frankenstein*. They're supposed to prevent sun damage to the mannequins, one with a white man-tailored shirt tucked into a grey A-line skirt and the other in a garish flowered housecoat with buttons the size of Rummoli chips, the same outfits from one year to the next. Pieces of cloth are tied around the mannequins' Styrofoam skulls, making them look like chemo patients. At their feet are limp purses with no crumpled paper to give them shape. There's a burgundy purse with zippers galore, a fake alligator, a black patent leather with an adjustable shoulder strap, and a few more.

Business hours aren't posted anywhere, but I assumed the store would open at 0900. In front of a *depanneur* across the street, I found a perfect vantage point to witness Miriam's arrival. 0900 came and went, then 1000. Still no sign of Miriam. At 1100, I went into a butcher shop to use the toilet and bought a baguette and a wedge of Havarti cheese. I had to take an OxyContin for my headache. I was shivering on a flimsy plastic chair, tearing hunks from the baguette in a long skinny paper bag when Miriam came into view, walking from the bus stop. It was 1150. I thought she'd get a ride or take a taxi. I concentrated on every detail. Her black trenchcoat, black stockings, black shoes, and black shoulder bag made her look like a box on peg legs. I could hear myself breathe excited little puffs of air on my way to her store.

Miriam was nowhere to be seen when I got there, so I flipped through a rack of pants and picked outs two pairs of bell-bottoms circa Sonny and Cher. God only knows how long they'd been hanging there. The black pair had a band of dust along the fold.

"You came back. *Barukh ha-shav.*" I was startled by Miriam's voice, looked up, and saw her standing under an Employees Only sign towards the back. She must have been watching me. Her eyes were twinkling.

"Hello Miriam, it's good to see you again. Yes, I came back."

As she walked toward me, I noticed her skirt was an empty cylinder, that she's broad across the chest, but her bottom half is shapeless.

"How have you been?"

"Not so very bad for my age." When she stood next to me, her petite stature was noticeable. She only came up to my chin.

There were no price tags on the merchandise, so I asked how much the black pants cost. She stroked the fabric and gave me her sales pitch. "Wool. Heavy weight," she said. "Very good quality slacks." That's what she called them, slacks. Something white was encrusted on her sweater, probably toothpaste. She was growing shabby along with the flare leg pants and the polyester blouses.

She tried to sell me a blazer, too. Called the two pieces "a pantsuit". I said I was only interested in the pants, so she agreed to let me buy them, but reluctantly, as if she were doing me a favour. She looked me straight in the eye and named a price that was higher than New Arrivals at The Gap, when most stores would've sent those ratty pants to Value Village years before. I bought them even though I had no intention of ever wearing them. I just wanted to prolong the conversation.

Miriam is more widely read than me, that's for sure. She was in the middle of an 800-page autobiography by Madeline Albright and asked me if I knew how bad it was for the Czechs during the war, which of course I didn't. She wouldn't have been impressed if I had told her I'd just finished *The Apprenticeship of Duddy Kravitz*.

On my second trip (or was it my third?), I noticed in *The Montreal Gazette* a public education series called *The Righteous*. I went to an Italian cultural centre to see a film, *Fifty Italians*, followed by the testimonial of a concentration camp survivor. "Testimonial" was the word the emcee used when she introduced the elderly man. As a child, he had been sheltered at a Catholic convent. At bedtime, the children were expected to brush their teeth, then file past Mother Superior and kiss a heavy silver cross in her hand. Then she blessed each of them. (I wondered if they were trying to convert all those little Jewish kids.) One young nun made a pet of him and told him it would be okay if he said a Jewish prayer under his blanket, so he did. It was a prayer his mother had taught him, "*Shema Yisrael.* Hear Israel, the Lord is our God . . . " Something like that.

The other event was at the Segal Centre. There were free appetizers (very fancy), some speeches, and a Klezmer trio playing what sounded like gypsy music to me. An award was presented to Carl Leblanc for *The Heart of Auschwitz*, supposedly a feel-good film. The presenter talked about a Nobel prize winner, Elie Wiesel, and said, "Never be a bystander to racism or intolerance." I'd never heard of Wiesel.

The next day, I went to a library. Most of the books were in French, but there was a small English section. Front and centre in a display of English books was *Hostage* by Elie Wiesel. It must've been placed there to catch my attention. It was too much of a coincidence. I skimmed through it and copied down an excerpt about Shabbat: "Joy predominates. Thank you God for giving us the most beautiful gift, the seventh day, so different from the others, a day whose peacefulness makes the trees and the stars in the sky sing." It was so beautiful. I didn't know much about Shabbat at the time, but who wouldn't wish for a day like that every week?

One of the times I went into Modern Apparel, Miriam was examining something cupped in the palm of a customer's hand. Miriam led her over to a wall of cardboard boxes I'd never noticed before. They were stacked to the ceiling, each with sample buttons glued to its end. Some had two, three, even four different sizes of the same button. The customer spotted a box with red buttons on a high shelf and pointed to it. "There it is. Would you like me to bring it down?"

"First you should know it will be one dollar for each button."

"No problem. I need two." She passed one box at a time to Miriam, working her way down from the top of the stack. When she reached the box with the red buttons, she put the rest back. Miriam opened the box and fished two buttons out of a plastic bag. "So these are the ones you want?"

"Yes. Perfect."

Miriam handed the box to the customer to place on the high shelf.

I was standing near the cash register, watching. While both of their backs were turned, I plucked Miriam's wallet from her purse left gaping on the counter. I don't know what got into me.

"My children, they don't like me to go anymore on ladders," Miriam said.

The customer paid the two dollars, thanked Miriam for her trouble, and left.

Miriam turned to me and said, "If she wasn't such a nice girl, I would've said 'No'. For two dollars it's not worth it."

I told her I was learning about Shabbat and asked if she'd ever heard of Elie Wiesel. "Pardon me," she said, so I repeated "Elie Wiesel" in a louder voice. She appeared to be lost in thought, then took in a deep breath, exhaled, and corrected my pronunciation of both "Elie" and "Wiesel". Obviously, she'd heard of him. Then she told me he's her cousin. I could hardly believe my ears. No way it could be coincidental — me hearing about him at the Segal Centre, one of his books practically pushed under my nose at the library, and then finding out he's Miriam's cousin.

On Fridays, Miriam closes early for Shabbat. She showed me a Chabad calendar with the time for sunset every Friday and Saturday. "You get these calendars from the bank. For free. Me, I'm not so strict." She tapped her head and chuckled. "I still have my hair." Her hair looked like she cut it herself, blunt, just below her ears. The dye she used could be called *Golden Brown Sugar*.

By this time, The Holocaust had wrapped itself around my leg and was forcing me to pay attention, so I decided to go to the museum called the Montreal Holocaust Memorial Centre on *Chemin de la Côte-Sainte-Catherine*. It has a glass showcase with the little heart-shaped birthday card that inspired Carl Leblanc's film. It's no bigger than my iPod. Some girls made the card in Auschwitz for their friend Fania, and she snuck it out in her armpit, which was incredibly brave.

I didn't know that Mackenzie King and his government turned a blind eye to Hitler's dirty business. On one of the archival documents, the name *Samuel Bronfman* leapt off the page. I must've gasped. During Prohibition, the wealthy Bronfman family used to store illegal whiskey in a vat in my grandparents' basement in Rhein, Saskatchewan. They thanked my grand-father for his trouble with a 1932 Ford Roadster, the first car in Rhein. It's the only scandal in my family history. I didn't know that some of the Bronfmans relocated from Saskatchewan to Montreal. The document said that when Canada refused to accept Jewish refugees, Samuel Bronfman offered to support five hundred Jewish children from Vichy France if Canada would accept them. The government pissed around making a decision until the children and their parents had been sent to the gas chambers.

When I asked Miriam if she'd ever visited the museum, she said, "Why would I go? Already I know it."

I listened to Elie Wiesel's Nobel Prize acceptance speech on YouTube. It was amazing. He's still alive and New York is his home.

One day, when I knew Miriam would be at the store, I went to her house. The address was in her wallet. I felt like a private eye, carrying a shoulder bag with my journal and camera. Her house is brick, two-storey, attached to other houses on both sides, probably close to a hundred years old, with a knee-high black wrought iron fence and gate. All the blinds were closed, so I couldn't see in, but I took photos of the outside. The lid of her mailbox was propped open and a pale blue Air Mail envelope was sticking out above other mail, so I pulled it out. There's a law about the privacy of mail, but I intended to return it. I was tempted to try one of the doors, but someone in the adjoining house might've caught me.

As for her wallet, she had cards for Quebec health insurance, Co-op Taxi, the Jewish Public Library, and an OPUS card for the bus and Metro, three twenty-dollar bills, some change, and an appointment card for Dr. R. B. Gelman, cardiologist. I kept the fuchsia clip-on earring I found in grains of sand in her zipper compartment. It's round and sparkly with six claws, looks like rhinestone. The only other thing I kept was her membership card for the National Council of Jewish Women of Canada, with her signature and home address. I didn't think she'd miss it. I returned the wallet to the Modern Apparel mailbox with *COBRA COCKER* graffiti spray-painted on it. On the way to the airport, I had the taxi driver swing past her house and I put the letter with the Jerusalem return address back in her mailbox. I had picked off the stamp, but couldn't bring myself to read it. .

Curtis says I've got a "Miriam Shrine". It takes up one corner of my desk. There are six pennies from her wallet (one for every time I visited Modern Apparel), a red button, a red maple leaf I picked from her backyard, the clip-on earring. (Must be a widowed earring, either that or something she found.) What else? Oh yeah, the swirl of golden brown sugar hairs on a folded Kleenex. (I used my thumb and index finger for tweezers and pulled out some of her hair caught under an upholstery tack on her chairback and tucked it into my glove. That was the day I got carried away. I also have the cash register receipt for the bell-bottoms and a Modern Apparel business card. I think that's all.

When I asked Miriam anything about the camp, most often she would insist, "I don't want to talk about the war." Then, without any prompting, she would say, "This one little thing I will tell for you."

Auschwitz in the diminutive. Push, pull. Close the door, open the door. Stay out, come in. Do up a button, undo it again.

I remember the date. It was November 7, the morning after Barack Obama was re-elected. The election, corruption, the Charbonneau Inquiry, mayors resigning — those were the topics of conversation at M. Bouchard's breakfast table. That was the last time I was at Modern Apparel.

Miriam said, "My sister, she's fair like you. I had to pinch her cheeks like so to make her look fit for work." Then she pinched both of her own cheeks. At that moment, I wanted to touch her. I wanted to pet her like a puppy, soothe the pinch-marks on her cheeks, but I didn't. Instead I squeezed her small hands. A quick squeeze, just long enough to feel her warmth. "I'll see you next year," I said, trying to sound cheery, but inside I was horrified. When she stretched up to pinch her cheeks, the sleeve of her sweater slipped down, and I saw the brand on her wrist. *12989.* My God! After the hand squeeze, she straightened her shoulders and walked away.

After I came home, things went to shit. I was suspended from Sunnyside after the pharmacist found the OxyContin count to be short. Sure, I helped myself to a few to relieve my pounding headaches. Three nurses, including me, had a key to the narcotics cabinet. Rosalie, our manager, reviewed the schedule and came to the conclusion that I was the common denominator. She confronted me and I resigned. I nixed the idea of a going-away tea. No way was I going to sit through a phony speech, a corsage, probably a skit with enema tubing cleverly conscripted to bring a laugh. They mailed me an engraved plaque. "With appreciation for nine years of dedicated service."

How do I spend my time now? Searching survivors' websites, renting movies (*Sophie's Choice, A Beautiful Life*), reading library books by Saul Friedlander and Primo Levi, plus all of Elie

Wiesel's. I know everything there is to know about *Kristallnacht* and The Stockholm Declaration of 2000. I track the trials of Nazi war criminals. You could say I've become an expert on the Holocaust. Curtis refers to it as my "project". He's putting the pressure on me to find another job. It's been eight months since my last time in Montreal.

A-1-1-2-9-8-9. I'm keeping a close eye on this pimply guy who calls himself an artist. I checked the public health inspectors' reports on every tattoo parlour before deciding on *Bizzart*.

Faith of My Father

I HAD A FATHER. TOGETHER, JUST the two of us, we waited for him to die. Like I mean how could I predict when he was gonna die? I'm not psychic. "Today's the day," I said. "God's gonna answer your prayer today. You're goin' to Heaven." I sell real estate for a living and for fun I drag an Arctic Cat snow machine on the grass, but I heard those words come outta my mouth. "Today's the day."

For years, Dad talked about dying. He insisted on goin' over his will and his funeral arrangements. "Remember, Faith, if you get a phone call telling you I died in my sleep, don't you cry. That's what I'm praying for, to be with my Lord and Saviour Jesus Christ and your mother and sister in Heaven."

I got fed up with it. "For Chrissake Dad, can't we talk about something a little more upbeat? Like what the McCains are fightin' about? Or one of them civil wars goin' on across the pond?"

"Now Faith, there's no need to take the name of the Lord in vain."

Honest, he'd deliver an entire sermon to a congregation of one, namely me. Take on the warbly voice of Jimmy Swaggart and quote Scripture passages warnin' me of eternal damnation if I didn't confess my sins and accept Jesus into my heart. He even paused for effect. I couldn't stand to listen no more, so I turned up the volume on his TV to drown him out, hope he'd take the hint. Tommy Hunter re-runs were my only salvation, no pun intended.

I heard the same speech over and over practically word-for-word. I'd have to go outside for a smoke so I wouldn't lose my patience with him. The longest I could stay was two nights . . . in a motel. He was a good father, always stood behind me, even when I screwed up.

That last time in his apartment, I asked him, "Wanna go to the buffet at Wongs? You said you were hungry for Chinese. Or we could order in."

"Oh, why don't you just heat up some chicken noodle soup for yourself? Crackers are in the corner cupboard. I haven't got much of an appetite. There's a can of Boost in the fridge, I'll have that."

I nearly puked when I seen that Boost with the dried pink scum in the holes punched with a can opener. Before I left, I gave him a hug at the door. On my way to the elevator, he called out, "I'll see you in Heaven, Faith." His benediction. I never even turned around.

We weren't one of them touchy-feely families, but after Mother died, I felt sorry for him and started hugging him when we'd say goodbye. It was awkward at first, but got to be a habit. An hour or so before it was time to leave, I'd get this acid in my stomach like that time Gerald ordered red-hot-and-spicy Thai curry. I'd keep on talkin', try to stay cheery, but it would fester until I had to rush to the bathroom and take a nervous shit. Sprayed the air with Lysol. I mean, a person can't help but wonder if it's the last time you're gonna see your old man when he's eighty-eight and has congestive heart failure.

When my parents named me Faith, they branded me. Their precious little girl was gonna be faith-filled, a church-goer, a God-fearer. How come boys don't get saddled with a name like Faith? There's even a hymn about men. *Faith of our Fathers, holy faith, we will be true to thee till death.* My name is a reminder that I let my parents down, thumbed my nose at destiny. So what's new? My kids let me down, too. One day it'll be my turn to sit in a seniors' apartment goin' over my life again and again, waitin' for my kids to phone or stop in. That is unless I wipe out in one of them snow machine Outlaw Shootouts. Line 'em up and knock 'em down. Go out in flames.

Him and Mother tried their best to brainwash me and Howard. Every Sunday morning we went to this Baptist church for two hours, one hour of Sunday School followed by another hour of church. And back to church in the evening for prayers and a gospel hymn sing. *Onward Christian Soldiers, marchin' as to war, with the cross of Jesus goin' on before.* We had to stay in our good clothes all day. There was barely time for three square meals, let alone doin' anything fun, unless my aunts and uncles and some of my cousins dropped by in the afternoon.

When I got home from the Grass Drags in the Annapolis Valley, there was a message from Home Care on my phone. Dad fell, so they put him in a nursing home in Sydney for one month. If some new medication got his blood pressure under control, he could go back to his apartment. A stroke, that must be what they were worried about. It barely sunk in at first because I was so pumped from besting the field in the Stock 700 on my F7. Big brass trophy in the back seat to prove it. And I got laid besides. Bonus!

Number 63 from Quebec took a shine to my machine, so I bragged up its performance. With the language barrier, I couldn't tell how much he understood, but he was definitely interested. Under his helmet were these moist black curls. He said something in French, then attempted a translation. "Can I ride you?"

A loud laugh poofed out of my mouth, but at the same time I could feel a pinch in my crotch. I was wearing a ruby BodyCover, one-piece with a full-length zipper, shows off my figure. I arched my back ever so slightly to draw his eye to my butt. He must've meant "Can I ride *with* you?" Or did he?

"Hop on, I'll take you for a run." He climbed on behind me and put his arms around my waist instead of grippin' the handles on either side of the machine. I took a scenic trail that cut through the valley. When I felt a hard bulge against my backbone, I knew what was comin' after the Awards Banquet. Lucky my period ended the day before.

Frenchie with the moist black curls from head to toe did not disappoint. A fiery meteor blasted through the sky toward earth and exploded in my feel-good place. And be damned if a second one didn't burst during the night. The way I look at it, what Dwayne don't know won't hurt him. My bad.

I called the nursing home and asked to speak to Herb Baron. I waited on the line for about ten minutes while someone brought him to the phone.

"Dad, are you okay?"

"Oh Faith, Faith, I never thought it would come to this. I never wanted to be in a nursing home. I fell when you were gone to one of them SkiDoo races. Don't remember what happened after that. I think this is gonna be the end for me." His voice was weak.

"I better come and see you."

"I don't know a soul here, don't even know the name of the place." There was a muffled conversation, then he came back on the line. "The nurse says it's the Cape Breton Care Centre, wherever that is. When you get to my age, you have to do what you're told."

"I'll be there as soon as I can."

I had a hard time convincin' anyone to cover my on-call shifts when I just came back from holidays. I updated my broker on Pending Offers to Purchase and potential new listings and headed out, trophy still in the back seat.

It was a five-hour drive. Kernels of memory popped in my brain, like the day I got my first bra and Mother said at the supper table, "Our little girl's all grown up." Tiger gettin' run over on the highway. A Sunday afternoon at Bras d'Or Lake when I was in a two-piece bathing suit racing my brother in the shallow water and some boys whistled at me. Stayin' out past my curfew and refusin' to get up Sunday morning.

When I landed my first job as a secretary in Halifax, I told them my name was Fay so they wouldn't think I was a Bible-thumper. I felt light, as if I'd shed a burden. Instead of Faith Baron, I was Fay Baron.

Later I became Fay Rakewich, then Fay Vogel. I picked some real losers, but a girl with buck teeth can't be choosy. I went back to my maiden name after Gerald divorced me, said all I cared about was work and money. That stung! I could've pointed out his (let's say) shortcomings, too. My birth certificate and passport are the only documents where the name Faith still appears. I won't be changin' my last name again, cross my heart and hope to die. A while back, when Dwayne got all hot and bothered about us living together, I was up front with him. "I'm not interested in gettin' married. Been there, done that. A couple times in fact. You can move into my condo and sleep with me, pay half the bills, but that's as far as I go." Don't sound very romantic, but it's worked out okay. Being with Dwayne is better than being by myself, but not much better.

The Care Centre smelled of bleach. I found Dad's room number in the directory on the wall. In the lounge, a TV was blarin', but all the old folks were sound asleep in their chairs. A whiteboard read: Today is Tuesday August 3. The weather is Sunny and Warm. The next meal is Supper.

I must've sounded like a team of horses clatterin' on that non-slip vinyl flooring in my bitch boots. A nurse at the desk glanced up at me but didn't say anything. Dad looked frail and pitiful sittin' in a little shoebox room. It was the first time I ever seen him in a wheelchair. The corners of his mouth curled into a little smile. "Faith," he said. He was the only person who still called me Faith.

We went to the common dining room for supper. Mushroom soup with a skin, a tunafish sandwich, a sweet pickle, and cherry Jello with a dab of Dream Whip. He ate a few bites, practically fell asleep at the table while I was tellin' him about his youngest great-grandson. I got this feeling he had given up. The other patients were slumped over their plates or had to be fed by one of the staff. Boy I could never work in a place with all females. Give me the world of men and I fit right in. At least you know where you stand.

I phoned Howard to tell him Dad was in the nursing home. It didn't seem to fizz on him. I must admit I found the place kinda interesting, even entertaining. The old babes with their perms looked like dried apple dolls, and the cronies wouldn't be able to find their way home in the dark, maybe not even in the daylight. This one guy shuffled up and down the hall callin', "Edna. Edna." After a while, it started to get on my nerves.

Dad fell asleep early and pretty soon I was noddin' off in the recliner. I took my boots off, pulled a blanket over myself, and slept right there in my clothes. I could've drove another half-hour to his apartment or got a motel room. On the way into town, I seen a motel with half-tons parked in a row and a sign that said "Take Out Rooms". Good for a chuckle.

In the mornin', they brought both of us breakfast trays, which I thought was real nice. Some woman kept callin' out "Nurse". They didn't get Dad dressed or take him to the bathroom, just put a pad under him. The head nurse said his heart was slowin' down and he was gettin' weaker. Readin' between the lines, she was tryin' to prepare me. I offered to pay for my meals.

I phoned my kids to tell them Dad was goin' downhill fast. Beth said she'd come on the weekend. She could sniff an inheritance.

Dad sat in bed propped up with pillows.

"I was just thinkin' about Uncle Ben," I said. "I bet he still goes out in that cape-style fishin' boat." I tried to make conversation, fill the silence, but he wasn't payin' attention. It's no wonder they call these places "God's waitin' room".

"Edna."

"Edna."

"Edna."

I thought I'd scream if I heard the name Edna one more time. When I went outside, I could've sworn I caught a whiff of two-stroke smoke, but there weren't no grass drags in the vicinity. The smell conjured up my romp with Frenchie.

I spent a second night on the recliner, woke up with a crick in my back. Should've got a motel room. The staff never brought no breakfast tray for Dad. Guess they decided he was pretty low. I took a facecloth and towel, sponge-bathed in the visitors' washroom, and put on clean underwear. I had an inkling Dad was going to die. After rehearsing in the washroom, I got up the courage to say, "Thanks . . . for . . . being . . . my . . . father . . . for . . . forty-five years." I choked on every word.

He said, "I've lived a long life, Faith. Eighty-eight years. And I'm a tired old man." Then he talked about the Jew at the general store in New Waterford, the town near the homestead shack with white-washed walls where he took his bride sixty years ago. "I have nothing to fear. I'm washed in the blood of the lamb." He was a shepherd makin' a last ditch effort to bring this lost sheep to the fold. I felt a prickle in the back of my neck and my tongue slid across my top teeth.

He dozed for an hour or more, then mumbled, "Horse manure."

"Pardon?"

"Horse manure. Heaven's just a bunch of horse manure."

Was he delirious? He was contradictin' what he preached his whole life. It gave me instant diarrhea. I rushed down the hall to the bathroom and, when I came back, he was asleep. I wanted to tell him, "Dad, those pills must be making you confused. Of course there's life after death. We'll all be reunited, it says so in the Bible, remember? There'll be glory and rejoicin' when you meet your Heavenly father."

"Edna."

"Edna."

I passed the afternoon on a hard chair readin' about multiday backcountry trips in a Sledworthy Magazine I found in my purse. I looked down at my spare tire and decided I shouldn't wear T-shirts with Spandex no more. I never put weight on my legs or ass, just around my middle, but not many women my age can squeeze into Size 10 jeans, so I guess I haven't gone to pot just yet.

Then it hit me that this was the end. I heard myself say, "Today's the day, Dad. God's gonna answer your prayer today. You're goin' to Heaven."

He managed to say "Faith" one last time. Then he was beyond talkin'. I was the only one with words.

"I'm sorry if I hurt you and Mother by changing my name." I sounded squeaky and timid.

His eyes were milky. Saliva flowed down from the corners of his mouth with no dentures. I watched his pulse throb in the folds of skin just above the top button of his pyjamas. His neck had these big ropey cords. My nose picked up talcum powder, medicine, damp must, and farts. The smells of an old man. Was he losin' consciousness?

Whenever he stirred, I told him, "I'm here with you," and offered him a sip of water with a bendable straw. I felt like a death coach.

I sat there all day with my childhood memories, like the time I overheard him say to my mother, "She'll never get a husband with those teeth." I could hardly wait till I was old enough to get the Hell out of that hick town, move to the city. After work on Fridays, Mary Jean and me used to go to the Lord Nelson for a beer and a cigarette. She was a chubby brunette with fluttery eyelashes and a pointy little nose like Veronica in the comics. One time I heard a guy at the next table say to his buddy, "Some gets the figure, some gets the face."

A nurse brought a tube of Vaseline and Q-tips to keep Dad's lips moist. Also a spoon and a turquoise plastic jug with ice chips. She told me they weren't goin' to get him up or give him anything by mouth.

"Edna."

"Edna."

That man had just been admitted on Tuesday and was lookin' for his wife, the nurse said. Poor bugger. I went out for a puff while she sponge-bathed Dad and changed his sheets. Then I sat on a chair pushed up against the bed sideways and held his hand. He lay still, with long spaces between breaths.

I was startled when a cat jumped up on his bed, but he didn't even stir. I shooed it away. Dad never liked cats.

Through the window, the sun was setting. My red nail polish was chipped. I'd have to do my nails before I showed up at work. That's what I was thinkin' when the feeling in the room shifted, like a stage play when the lighting changes and you know something important is gonna happen. Dad grew paler and dimmer until he was see-through. So help me God, if you put a candle behind him, you could've seen his veins and his organs. It was as if his flesh softened into candle wax. I held his hand, cool and smooth as satin, and said, "I love you Dad" for the first and last time. His eyes opened wide like he was flabbergasted, and stayed that way. Then he stopped breathin'. I waited for the next breath, but it didn't come. He kept on starin'. I swear his spirit was sucked right out of his body and rose into the great beyond. Then his eyes closed. That was it, he was dead.

I untangled my hand from his and looked at my wristwatch. It was ten o'clock. There weren't no lights on. It was dark inside and out. Now here's the weirdest part. His body started to glow a yellowish colour. I seen a program on the Discovery Channel about corpses givin' off phosphorescence. That must've been what was happenin'. It only lasted a few seconds. I stayed sittin' on the chair and laid my cheek down on his chest. I was an orphan. That's when the tears came. I fell asleep. Dad and I slept together until a nurse escorted Beth and her husband Jeremy into the room. The nurse stopped in the doorway and let out a little gasp. Beth started to sob. "We should've come sooner. I wanted to say goodbye to Pa."

The nurse asked if a cat came into Dad's room. She said it always pays a visit to residents on the day of their death.

Jeremy called me over to the window to look at the northern lights. They were green, churning in the sky above the nursing home. He said they were so spectacular that him and Beth pulled over onto the shoulder of the highway to watch them, even though they were in a hurry. That was two hours earlier, at ten o'clock.

The next week was a blur. Cleanin' out Dad's apartment, puttin' in an appearance at work, a lot of drivin'. Dwayne was a real sweetheart, bought me flowers, took time off work, helped haul stuff to the dump, held my hand at the funeral even though he never met Dad. I didn't know he had it in him.

The Baptist minister said Dad had a strong faith. Whenever he said the word "faith", naturally my ears perked up. Dad gave me the gift of his last word, but with strings attached. Faith, my Christian name.

I witnessed my father passin' from life to death, and it blew me away. It was even better than my childhood book of Bible stories, the picture of a team of flyin' white horses pullin' a chariot across the sky to a castle on puffy clouds, and God in a white robe waitin' on a street paved in gold. Dad's spirit left his body and was escorted to Heaven, if there is such a place, by the northern lights. When I Googled "aurora borealis" and skimmed over the big words, I found out Indians think northern lights are the dance of the spirits.

It's gonna be a year this month since Dad passed on. The housing market is hot, so I'm makin' a good chunk of change. I buggered up my leg when I sideswiped a tree over at Keji, so I have to sit out the grass drags this season.

A few times Dad has come in the night sky to visit me. I was showin' a property and went outside for a smoke so my clients could talk in private. At first there was just a flicker off in the distance. I turned and saw it fan out like an accordion, mostly white-ish. I felt a prickle in the back of my neck, and my tongue slid across my top teeth. It didn't last long, but I knew it was Dad. I had to rush inside to the bathroom.

Dwayne and me took a week of holidays in July. He rented a little cabin at Lake Deception, called it romantic. It was pretty basic, but I didn't complain. One night he made us a campfire and we sipped on a couple brew. The sky was pitch black except for stars, and the northern lights were purple and green. "I'm doin' okay Dad," I said under my breath. Dwayne doesn't know my father is what's called a celestial being, but I've seen the proof of it.

Ten Reasons To Blame Your Mother

Because she married your father.
Because she didn't marry your father.
Because she was never at home.
Because she was always at home.
Because she never made dinner.
Because she made you come home for dinner.
Because she was overprotective.
Because she failed to protect you.
Because she left your father.
Because she didn't leave your father.

Acknowledgements

With my thanks to . . .

Thistledown Press for sending my work out into the world,

The Saskatchewan Arts Board for two Independent Artists' Grants,

The Banff Centre, St. Peter's College, the Saskatchewan Writers' Guild, and The Munster Literature Centre (Cork, Ireland) for educational opportunities,

Connie Gault, for introducing me to Short Fiction during the 2009 Saskatchewan Writers' Guild Mentorship Program,

Seán Virgo, for extending invitations for me to imagine scenes more fully ,

Sarah Selecky, Jessica Grant, Lynda Monahan, Dave Margoshes, and Yvette Nolan for generously sharing their knowledge and experience,

Prairie Quills, my writers' group in Swift Current, Saskatchewan,

Elizabeth Withey, my daughter and writing comrade,

James Worrell, my love.

Versions of the following stories have been published previously:

"A Bit of Bother", *Spring* 2013

"Mary Had a Lamb", the *Nashwaak Review* 2012

"Lunch At The Empire State Building", the *Prairie Journal* online 2012

"Liam the Leprechaun"(excerpt from "Mary Had a Lamb") broadcast on CBC Radio SoundXchange 2012

"Four Fridays", *Mental Munching*, Prairie Quills Anthology 2012

"Foul Play Not Suspected", Brighton UK Community of Writers online 2010

"Big Mary's Love Life" ("Mary Had a Lamb"), *Characters*, Prairie Quills Anthology, 2008

The lyrics on page 106 are by Connie Kaldor excerpted from "Maria's Song (Batoche)" from the album *Grocery Moonlight* (Coyote Entertainment, 1984).

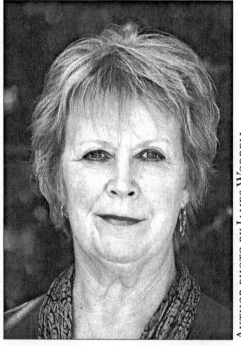

Author photo by James Worrell

P. J. Worrell has studied with Sarah Selecky, Connie Gault, Jessica Grant, Seán Virgo, Lynda Monahan, and Michele Roberts as mentors. She has enjoyed modest success in the world of publication and contests. Social work practice in mental health and geriatrics have provided fodder for her stories. She has one foot in Swift Current, Saskatchewan and the other in a cabin at a northern lake.